Dr. Jensen's
NUTRITION
HANDBOOK

Dr. Jensen's NUTRITION HANDBOOK

A DAILY REGIMEN FOR HEALTHY LIVING

Bernard Jensen, D.C., Ph.D.
Clinical Nutritionist

KEATS PUBLISHING

LOS ANGELES

NTC/Contemporary Publishing Group

The purpose of this book is to educate. It is sold with the understanding that the publisher and author shall have neither liability
nor responsibility for any injury caused or alleged to be caused
directly or indirectly by the information contained in this book.
While every effort has been made to ensure its accuracy, the book's
contents should not be construed as medical advice. Each person's
health needs are unique. To obtain recommendations appropriate to
your particular situation, please consult a qualified health-care provider.

Library of Congress Cataloging-in-Publication Data

Jensen, Bernard, 1908–
    [Nutrition handbook]
    Dr. Jensen's nutrition handbook : a daily regimen for
  healthy living / Bernard Jensen.
        p. cm.
    Includes index.
    ISBN 0-658-00278-3
      I. Nutrition. 2. Health. I. Title: Doctor Jensen's
    nutrition handbook. II. Title.
    RA784. J457 2000
    613.2—dc21   99-058505

Design by Andrea Reider
Illustrations by Ilene Robinette, Ilene Robinette Studio

Published by Keats Publishing
A division of NTC/Contemporary Publishing Group, Inc.
4255 West Touhy Avenue, Lincolnwood (Chicago), Illinois 60712, U.S.A.

Printed in the United States of America

International Standard Book Number: 0-658-00278-3

00 01 02 03 04 VP 18 17 16 15 14 13 12 11 10 9 8 7 6 5 4 3 2 1

*To my brothers and sisters all over the world
who seek the best in life, physically, mentally,
and spiritually, and who realize that nutrition wisdom
is one of the essential keys to achieving their goal.*

CONTENTS

INTRODUCTION

There is a good deal of confusion today about nutrition. We should be concerned about what we are consuming. Most people, however, have little understanding of what the body is made from or what it needs. People build a body chemistry on the kinds of foods they eat; therefore, the body is only as healthy as the kinds of foods that are put in it. The way we are living and eating will determine our future. Certainly, self-care should be an important part of our daily lives. Hippocrates said, "Let your food be your medicine, and your medicine be your food." He also said that the doctor of the future will never understand disease until he understands the makeup of food. Nutrition in our time is being accepted in the context presented by Hippocrates in his time.

There is much research being conducted today on contributing factors to illness and disease, and why many diseases are increasing in the population. Some alarming statistics follow. An estimated 35 percent of all cancer deaths may be linked to diet. Many people treated with drugs have developed iatrogenic illnesses. *Taber's Cyclopedic Medical Dictionary* (Philadelphia: F. A.

Davis Company, 1997) defines iatrogenic disease/disorder as "any adverse mental or physical condition induced in a patient through the effects of treatment by a physician or surgeon." The term implies that such effects could have been avoided by proper and judicious care on the part of the physician. An unknown number of people suffer from diseases and disturbances brought on by environmental pollution and chemical pollutants in the workplace and in the home. Forty million people in this country now have allergies. More than fifty billion nonprescription pain relief tablets were sold in 1998. Sixty-two million people suffer from digestive disorders. It has been found that one out of every three deaths is from heart disease, and one out of four deaths in 1998 was due to cancer. Fifteen percent of the population have some form of arthritis. In addition, 63 percent of our teenagers failed to meet minimum recommended standards for vigorous exercise three times weekly. It is my opinion that it is time for us to meet these problems head-on and bring up the health level of our nation.

A medical study of the development of cardiovascular disease turned up six primary risk factors. They are obesity, hypertension, elevated cholesterol levels, diabetes, smoking, and lack of exercise. All but the last two are seriously affected by what we eat. I feel that many Americans have grossly underestimated the power of foods to keep themselves disease-free, energetic, and at a peak level of wellness. Eating right should start with our children.

I have spent many years of research in order to be able to put food ideas into an orderly program. I have attempted to present food concepts in a simple, practical way so that people can better understand how to properly nourish their bodies. Confusion about nutrition encourages people to listen to repetitious commercials and be persuaded by them. The worst thing about so many of the packaged food products on the market today is that they are not developed by dietitians, doctors, nutritionists, or people with suitable nutritional training. In 1997, the per capita health-care cost was a little under $4,000. Scientific reports are telling us that a well-balanced diet, enriched with fruits, vegetables, and grains and low in fat, sugar, and salt, significantly lowers the risks for developing heart disease, cancer, osteoporosis, arthritis, and other degenerative diseases.

A spokeswoman for the National Food Processors Association said that food labels should communicate facts and not educate. I agree with her, but I also feel that people need a nutritional education program that is uncomplicated, easy to understand, and simple to put into practice. Many people are asking questions about what kinds of foods are best to eat. Should we eat grains? Is meat good for us? Should we leave out milk entirely? Do we need salt?

I have developed a nutritional program that will support all body structures, restore nutrient-depleted tissues, repair damaged tissues, and rejuvenate the energy production capability of the cells of the body. I have found that the brain needs certain nutrients, the glands need other kinds of food, and the bones need still others. If we neglect feeding any system in the body, any organ of the body, that system or organ can become so depleted that its ability to function is severely impaired. Every organ, gland, tissue, and system has to be fed so it can keep functioning normally. This book describes a simple, step-by-step, practical program I have developed over many years to help guide my patients into a healthy lifestyle and to ensure that they know how to meet the nutritional requirements of their bodies for the best possible health.

CHAPTER 1

RECOMMENDED DAILY FOOD PROGRAM

M y healing food laws are presented in this chapter. By following these eleven laws, you will meet your basic needs for sufficient intake of calories, enzymes, vitamins, minerals, protein, carbohydrates, and lipids. Always remember the importance of foods as described in these laws. Our health is determined as much by what we don't eat as by what we do eat. A defective diet can cause nutritional deficiencies that lead to future disease. If we neglect vegetables, for example, we prevent our bodies from receiving needed chemical elements, enzymes, and fiber. Lack of sufficient proteins, carbohydrates, and fats can impair body functions, as can insufficient amounts of vitamins, minerals, and trace elements. All of these have to be considered.

I believe there are three basics that lead to disease. First are the *inherent weaknesses* we inherit from our parents. Second are the *toxic substances* we accumulate in our bodies from environmental pollution, chemicals at work or home, residues of drugs, food additives, and metabolic wastes retained in the body. Third are the *chemical deficiencies* we develop in the body due to an inadequate diet or digestive problems. My food program is designed to help the body overcome these weaknesses. It will help build the immune system as well as strengthen the inherent weaknesses, gradually remove the toxins stored in the body, and replace the deficient biochemicals. The foods I recommend will nourish the body with sufficient nutrients to restore chemical balance and supply the minerals and trace elements needed by depleted tissues.

DR. JENSEN'S FOOD LAWS

Law No. 1: As Much As Possible, Eat Natural, Pure, Whole, and Fresh Foods

If you would like to develop a healthy body, abundant energy, and a strong immune system, focus on foods that are *natural, pure, whole,* and *fresh.* "Natural" means that the foods should be organically grown, without exposure to insecticides or chemical sprays, in mineral-rich soil that contains all the nutrients necessary for the healthy growth of the plants. Foods must be "pure" without chemical additives, salt, or sugar. "Whole" means that no nutritionally valuable part of the food should be removed; for example, cereal grains such as wheat or rice should be whole, not with the outer hull milled off. (Barley is an exception. The two outer husks are inedible and must be milled off.) Potatoes, carrots, apples, and other fruits and vegetables with edible skins should be eaten with the skins. (Obviously, there are exceptions like avocados, pineapples, citrus, bananas, nuts, and so on.) No refined foods should be used. Foods are considered "fresh" if they would normally spoil or lose significant nutritional value if they were stored. Fruits, berries, lettuce, spinach, and broccoli are examples of foods that should be eaten fresh to get the most nutritional value from them. This law implies that packaged, processed, or manufactured foods (which are no longer natural, pure, whole, or fresh) should be avoided.

In nature, foods contain groups of vitamins, minerals, enzymes, and other nutrients that work synergistically when all are eaten together in a whole food. If anything is added or removed, the synergy is disrupted. Synergy means something like "mutually enhancing." When wheat is milled, twenty-two nutrients are greatly reduced. The refining process also removes fiber, lignins, phytophenolic acids, and phytoestrogens, all of which enhance health in various ways and are believed to reduce the risk of heart disease, cancer, and diabetes. (A Harvard University study of nurses found that the nurses with the lowest fiber intake and the highest sugary/starchy-food intake showed more than a twofold increase in diabetes over those who used more fiber and less sugary/starchy foods.)

Most doctors believe that refined sugar triggers hyperactivity in a certain percentage of children, mostly boys. Hyperactive kids are more active and sometimes unruly, with short attention spans and a tendency to act impulsively. In the 1970s, foods containing salicylates were suspected of causing hyperactivity and attention deficit disorder. Dr. Benjamin F. Feingold highlighted salicylate-containing foods as the villains in his book *Why Your Child Is Hyperactive* (New York: Random House, 1975), and encouraged parents of hyperactive children to put them on a no-salicylate diet. Thousands of parents swore that the diet worked wonders with their children. However, double-blind studies by food scientists didn't confirm Dr. Feingold's claims. In the studies, hyperactive children on no-salicylate diets didn't improve. Some experts felt that as parents worked with the Feingold diet, it was the attention given to their children that brought the improvement, not the diet itself. I personally feel that a balanced diet will help most hyperactive children.

Foods high in white sugar should be avoided entirely. If one eats any sweets at all, they should come from nature. Fruits have plenty of sugar. Dried fruits, such as dates, figs, prunes, and raisins, make a wonderful dessert high in iron. A little raw honey or true maple syrup occasionally will not hurt. Sixty years ago, we consumed an average of 16 pounds of sugar per person in the United States annually. In 1997, Americans averaged 154.1 pounds of sugar per person. This is far too much.

When I go into a restaurant, I sometimes see people adding salt to their foods before they even taste it. If a person has used salt for years, their taste buds have become insensitive and they use more and more salt to be able to taste it. Athletes who sweat profusely may lose as much as ten to twelve pounds of water in a professional game. They would benefit from using sun-evaporated sea salt to replace salt loss from perspiration. However, I feel that refined table salt (which is pure sodium chloride and often contains an aluminum compound) should be avoided entirely. Nature provides us with plenty of organic sodium in fresh vegetables and fruit to meet normal require-ments. Sodium in this natural form is necessary to our health.

Coffee, most soft drinks, and chocolate (which are high in caffeine) should be eliminated from the diet. Caffeine is a strong stimulant to the heart and nervous system. It has no nourishment value at all. Alcohol is toxic in large amounts and is hard on the liver. The body has to use vital nutrients and energy in order to detoxify the alcohol, which destroys cells by desiccation as it circulates and as it is broken down. In many restaurants and bars, notices are posted warning pregnant women of fetal alcohol syndrome caused by consumption of alcohol during the development stages of the fetus. When the body is balanced with all the nutrients it needs, it will not have such a craving for sugar, salt, caffeine, or alcohol.

Chocolate, one of the favorite snack and dessert foods of people in many countries, is also usually near the top of any doctor's list of food allergens. Chocolate is made from cocoa beans that are ground up into a paste that is about 50 percent fat. Chocolate contains caffeine and theobromine, both of which speed up the heartbeat and stimulate the central nervous system. Among the problems some people have with chocolate are migraine headaches, abdominal pain, asthma attacks, and eczema. Chocolate contains bioamines similar to histamine that can stimulate allergy-like reactions that are not true allergies. Some health scientists believe that the bioamines in chocolate can aggravate existing arthritis inflammation and pain.

Most foods that are not natural, pure, whole, and fresh should be avoided. We should also avoid fried foods, fatty foods, white rice, pasteurized milk products, and white flour, which is low in nutrients and high in gluten. (Gluten is the substance in wheat and other grains that causes dough to stick together.) A chemical in gluten causes celiac disease by destroying villi in the wall of the small intestine. Celiac disease is an intestinal malabsorption syndrome characterized by diarrhea, weight loss, bleeding tendency, and extreme malnutrition. The only known treatment of this disease is a strict gluten-free diet that avoids all products made of wheat, oats, barley, and rye. This diet may have to be continued for an indefinite period.

The average American consumes 27 percent of their diet in cow's milk products. This is far too much. Milk substitutes derived from raw nuts or seeds, soybeans, or rice can replace cow's milk in your diet. I personally prefer using fresh goat's milk. Besides its pleasant taste, it is close to human milk. It nourishes the nervous system and glands and is more easily digested than cow milk because its fat particles are smaller. I have seen a few of my patients virtually revived from near-death conditions with fresh, warm goat's milk. Goat's milk is surely a vitality-producing food. I am also pleased to find soy milk, rice milk, and almond milk on the shelves of natural food stores and some supermarkets.

If you were to study the digestive and assimilative functions of the human body, you would gain a better understanding of the importance of foods being natural, whole, fresh, and pure. Our bodies are designed to utilize certain foods well but cannot make healthy tissue from foods not up to par. When the body becomes deficient in certain chemical elements, the symptoms of scurvy, beriberi, or other diseases may occur. Sailors at sea experienced these centuries ago and began to take citrus fruits and whole grains with them on their journeys. Often, whole countries can be affected, such as those nations far from the sea whose people suffer from goiter, an iodine-deficiency disease.

I believe there isn't a disease in which the person does not have mineral shortages and dietary deficiencies, either as contributing factors to developing the disease or as consequences of the disease ravaging certain tissues. The best way to be sure we get all the nutrients we need to be healthy is to eat foods that are as close as possible to the way nature provides them—fresh, whole, natural, and pure.

Law No. 2: Sixty Percent of the Foods We Eat Should Be Raw

I believe that raw foods contain living enzymes that help protect and preserve the vitamins and minerals in those foods. Heat, air, and contact with water (boiling) greatly reduce the vitamin and nutrient content of foods. In cooking foods by boiling, 48 percent of the iron is lost, 31 percent of the calcium is destroyed, 46 percent of the phosphorus is wasted, and 45 percent of the magnesium is boiled away. Vitamin C and B-complex vitamins are reduced or destroyed by cooking. Some nutritionists advise consuming 100 percent raw foods; however, I feel that this approach is quite extreme and would be very difficult for most people to follow. I believe that if 60 percent of the diet is raw, that's sufficient.

The raw egg yolk is one of the best sources of protein one can consume. Reports say that eggs are high in cholesterol. (A large chicken egg has 274 milligrams of cholesterol.) However, lecithin, which helps keep cholesterol in the bloodstream, is 21 percent, by weight, of the yolk. If the egg is not overheated, the lecithin will keep the cholesterol safely in solution in the blood. An egg has all the nutrients necessary to build a new life. It is a wonderful drink that is high in iron and a great tonic for the nerves.

Raw seeds and nuts are relatively high in lecithin, protein, and vitamin E, and are excellent foods for the nerves and glands. Nuts are good sources of protein, unsaturated fats, B-complex vitamins, vitamin E, calcium, iron, copper, and magnesium.

Seeds contain many of the same nutrients, plus zinc and fluorine. Seed and nut butters are delicious additions to soups and salads. Seeds and nuts help protect the heart and may have anticancer properties.

Raw fruits are high in bioflavonoids, which are necessary for healthy connective tissues in the skin, veins, and capillaries. Bioflavonoids are water-soluble substances composed of rutin, citrine, hesperidine, flavones, and flavonols. I believe they help prevent wrinkles, varicose veins, and hemorrhoids (which are caused by straining the gut tissue in the rectum).

Raw green vegetables, especially leafy greens, are high in chlorophyll, which is nature's best internal cleanser. Chlorophyll and hemoglobin are similar in molecular structure except that hemoglobin has an iron atom whereas chlorophyll has a magnesium atom. Raw yellow and green vegetables are high in beta-carotene (pro-vitamin A), an antioxidant that helps prevent free radicals from damaging tissue.

Chewing raw foods well helps to develop good teeth, healthy gums, and strong jaws. Be sure to chew your food about thirty-two times each bite so that you will receive the maximum benefit from it. Eat plenty of raw vegetables, nuts, seeds, and fruits from Mother Nature's bounteous table each day to build a healthy, happy body.

Law No. 3: Balance Your Body Chemistry with 80 Percent Alkaline Foods and 20 Percent Acid Foods

Close to 80 percent of the nutrients carried in the blood are alkaline and about 20 percent are acid. To help keep the blood at the right acid–alkaline balance (pH 7.4), I use an easy-to-remember rule of thumb. I have found that six vegetables and two fruits make up the 80 percent alkaline foods we need, while one protein and one starch make up the 20 percent acid foods, when the proper portions are used. What are proper portions? For men, 60 grams of protein, and for women, 45 grams. The starches (grain, potatoes, squash) should be about 80 grams. The vegetables and fruits should total around 220 grams, ideally, of alkaline foods.

Proteins and many starches are acid-forming, and nearly all the metabolic wastes of the body are acidic. We need alkaline-forming foods, such as fruit and vegetables, so that their alkaline salts (potassium, sodium, calcium, magnesium, and so on) will neutralize the acid wastes. We should recognize that the fresher the food, the more alkaline it is. The longer it is kept, the more acid it becomes.

Meats contain uric acid and should be eaten sparingly. Uric acid may contribute to high blood pressure, gout, arthritis, urinary tract disorders, and many other problems. People who suffer from too much uric acid in the body have eaten too much acid-forming meat and not enough alkaline-forming salads. There is no reason we should add to the acid conditions in our body by including too much acidic food as found in proteins and starches. In my experience, acid waste not properly disposed of is the cause of many disturbances, health problems, and diseases.

Law No. 4: Consume Six Vegetables, Two Fruits, One Starch, and One Protein Daily

During my many years of active sanitarium practice and teaching over 300,000 patients and students with various health problems, I worked out these proportions as being the most beneficial for providing all the nutrients the body needs on a daily basis. This arrangement can be used for all ages; however, the diet of children can be altered to include two starches and one protein daily, with smaller portions than adults. For those who are over the age of forty, their diet may work better with two proteins and one starch daily. This may be regulated according to the physical demands for nutritional support and energy. Juices or herbal teas can be taken between meals.

Vegetables are high in fiber and minerals. Fruits are high in natural, complex sugars and vitamins. Starch is for energy and protein is for cell repair and upkeep, especially of the brain and nerves.

Remember, it is important to eat 80 percent of the alkaline foods daily and 20 percent of the acid foods daily. Six vegetables plus two fruits make up the 80 percent alkaline proportion. One starch plus one protein will make up the 20 percent acid proportion. When you eat these amounts, you will have balanced proportions of acid and alkaline foods as well as all the fiber and nutrients your body needs to be healthy.

Most nutritionists believe we should have a certain "window" of total carbohydrates each day, from 100 to 300 grams, and I agree. By eating the right foods in the proportions I have listed, you will get all the trace elements you need each day.

Eating a variety of vegetables is important, especially the cruciferous vegetables, which are members of the mustard family, like broccoli and cabbage. Researchers have found that they are very helpful in preventing cancer. These high-sulfur foods also help to develop lecithin, which is a dissolver of hardening in the arteries and cholesterol excess. A review of 156 studies published in the *Journal of Nutrition and Cancer* showed that in 128 of the studies, fruits and vegetables offered significant protection against cancers of the lungs, colon, breast, cervix, esophagus, oral cavities, stomach, pancreas, and ovaries. Greens are wonderful for building up the iron in the body. They are a tonic for anemics because iron is a key component in building hemoglobin. Iron attracts oxygen, and these two elements give us energy to work with.

Calcium is found in seeds, nuts, beans, legumes, greens, and grains as well as milk and milk products. Children and young people need more calcium than people who are over thirty because they are building bone. Some people get all their calcium from milk products. We can become anemic if we lean too much on milk products in our food regimen because milk products lack iron. Milk is notorious for developing unwanted mucus and catarrh in some people.

For the vegetables and fruits, I recommend those that are fresh, organically grown, and fully ripe, when possible. For your daily starch requirement, choose from whole grains such as rice, rye, millet, oats, barley, and yellow cornmeal. Any of these can be cooked as a hot cereal with soy, rice, nut, or seed milk over them.

Avoid wheat and wheat products, or minimize them in your diet. Many people have allergies to wheat because Americans have used wheat products to excess. Bread usually contains yeast and is not good for those with digestive troubles or *Candida albicans*.

For your protection, choose your proteins from nuts, seeds, legumes, soft-boiled eggs, raw goat's milk or cheese, fish, or meat from organically fed poultry or livestock. One may have fish three times a week and meat once or twice a week. The king of the nuts is the almond because it is the alkaline nut that rates highest in overall nutritional content. The king of the seeds is the sesame, which is very high in calcium. The easiest to digest of the legumes is the lentil. If you prefer to be a vegetarian, you can acquire all your protein from nuts, seeds, grains, and legumes.

Law No. 5: Eat a Variety of Foods Every Day

It is important to eat a variety of foods each day to ensure taking in a wide variety of nutrients. Some people like to eat mostly potatoes; others like to eat only meat. Eating only a few foods or the same foods every day creates a high risk of nutritional deficiencies. When we look at the intricate chemical makeup of the body, we can see it is composed of different kinds of vitamins, minerals, and other nutrients. Within the body is an entire universe of simultaneous and interactive functions. This is why I stress the importance of eating a wide variety of foods that are whole, pure, natural, and fresh. If we eat these kinds of foods in variety, we can be more confident that our diet contains all the vital elements needed by the body to be healthy, strong, and vibrant.

I feel that a healthy way of living and eating is certainly the most important physical priority in life. Our bodies are made from the dust of the earth, and our bones need different nutrients than our muscles. The adrenal gland has a different makeup than the thyroid gland. Our lungs need nutrients different from those our eyes need.

Often, people do not have an adequate understanding of the connection between health and nutrition. They do not understand why they should incorporate a wide variety of foods in their diet on a daily basis, so they turn to fad diets. There are so many special diets being offered as solutions to the overweight problems that exist today. There are many reducing diets, such as carrot juice diets, protein diets, rice diets, and the Beverly Hills diet. People are looking for a quick fix for their weight problems. We find that, even with all the dietetic programs we have today, very few people actually have a healthy way of living. When people follow very limited diets, often they have not considered the various needs of all body systems and tissues. If the body is not fed right, it will not work right.

There are numerous misconceptions of what makes a good food. People believe they have to measure food by calories, not realizing that 160 grams of spinach containing only 37 calories has more nutritional value than the same amount of pecan pie containing 670 calories! It is the *quality* of a food that is important. We need a certain amount of calories to run the body properly, but the calories should come from a wide variety of nutrient-dense foods that are pure, whole, natural, and fresh. When we eat the right kinds of foods, they will balance the body chemistry, the health level will improve, and weight will become normalized.

If you want to lose weight, follow my healthy way of eating and cut down the size of your portions for one month or longer. The amount you eat determines the weight you will have. Watch your fat intake, eat garden salads with lunch and dinner, cut down your meat and starch intake, don't add butter to your cooked vegetables, eat more vegetables, and go easy on the salt. This is the healthy way to diet. This program is half eliminating and half building.

Fad diets may take the weight off for a short period of time, but this doesn't last when the person returns to their old way of eating. A rice diet or a carrot juice diet *may* improve one's health for a time, but if a person has not learned a new way of living and eating and they return to the lifestyle that caused the problem in the first place, the old weight will come back.

So we must eat a variety of foods that are pure, natural, whole, and fresh. Proper nutrition can help prevent atherosclerosis, cancer, and other degenerative ailments. Atherosclerosis can be produced from a lack of organic sodium, which keeps the veins and arteries soft and pliable. We must have potassium for the heart muscle. We need organic sodium and vitamin B_6 to keep the joints loose and limber. The pancreas needs silicon to be healthy, and the thyroid needs iodine. We must have certain foods and the nutrients contained within those foods to keep all the functions of the body working properly.

In studying the colors of foods, you will find that each color has a different effect on the body. Red is an arterial stimulant. Cayenne pepper brings up the circulation and improves the digestion. Green is healing. Green foods are sedatives and can help us to be more relaxed. Practically all vegetables and fruits that are considered laxative in nature are yellow and orange. I teach my students to eat a "rainbow" salad containing a variety of colorful vegetables and thus a variety of nutrients.

I have taught my students to "know your sevens," in order to help them have a variety of foods each day. Know seven good salads, seven good salad dressings, seven good proteins, and seven good starches. Try to work out the variety to the best of your ability, then learn more than seven; try fourteen, so you can increase your variety of foods.

Law No. 6: Separate Starches and Proteins

Try to separate starches and proteins, eating them at different meals. One reason for this is that starches are digested by the enzyme amylase (which is alkaline), and proteins are digested mostly by hydrochloric acid, pepsin, and trypsin (which are acidic). If the stomach contains both starches and proteins, both types of enzymes will be attempting to digest the food, but they do not work well together because one is alkaline and the other acidic. This can lead to indigestion, with the starches fermenting and the meat, chicken, or fish proteins putrefying. Another reason I advocate separating starches and proteins to different meals is because people tend to fill up on "meat and potatoes," and eat fewer vegetables. I have seen people not get the vitamins and minerals they need because they are not eating the fruit and vegetables served at the same meal. If a person is ill or has a digestive disorder, then they need to be more conscientious about food separation. Separating starches and proteins assists the body in efficient digestion.

I recommend that you have your proteins and starches at different meals, not because they don't digest well together, but so you will be able to eat more fruits and vegetables at each meal. People tend to fill up on protein and starch, then neglect their vegetables. I want you to have several vegetables with each meal for your health's sake; when you are hungry, they taste wonderful.

There are poor food combinations, and I will mention a few. Dried fruits do not mix well with fresh fruits. Unless dried fruits have been reconstituted and brought back to their natural state, it is best not to eat them, unless you drink a glass of water as you eat them. It is best not to have grapefruit and dates together. Dried fruits should be reconstituted by putting the dried fruit in a pan of cold water the evening before they are to be eaten. Bring them to a boil, let the water boil for about three minutes, then turn off the heat and let them soak overnight. Melon should be eaten by itself, at least half an hour apart from any other food. It is best to have your fruit at breakfast and at 3 P.M. See chapter 2 for suggested menus.

There are various opinions about having liquids with meals. I believe having ice-cold drinks with meals interferes with digestion. Another thought is that the additional water in liquids will dilute the digestive enzyme concentration in the small intestine and reduce the enzymes' ability to break down the food particles.

One should eat a starch food along with a salad at lunch or supper (for example, a salad and a baked potato) or a protein, a salad, and some steamed vegetables at the other meal on the same day (for example, broiled fish, salad, and steamed broccoli). These menus can be used for lunch or dinner. One should always eat a raw salad with a heavy starch, such as potatoes, or with a protein in order to integrate the fiber from the salad with the starch or protein. The purpose is to sustain a healthy bowel transit time, which reduces cholesterol reabsorption through the bowel wall and carries off more fats.

I believe there is an age range when many people need more protein or more starches. During the first twenty years of life, when young persons are very active and the body is busy building tissue, there is a greater need for starches, vegetables, and fruits. From twenty to fifty years of age, when people are less physically active, perhaps using their minds more, there is a greater need for proteins. Proteins support and sustain the brain and nervous system, as do the cholesterol and lecithin associated with some proteins (such as eggs). Throughout our lives, we should think about matching our dietary intake with what is taking place in each particular season of life.

Law No. 7: Include Sufficient Fiber in the Diet

It was Dr. Denis Burkitt's pioneering studies in the 1960s with East African rural natives that brought the value of fiber to the attention of our nation's medical community and the public at large. Dr. Burkitt had discovered that heart disease, colon cancer, diverticulosis, appendicitis, hemorrhoids, and constipation were almost nonexistent in natives whose diet consisted largely of high-fiber cereals, while the same diseases were common among the British living in the same area. Dr. Burkitt noted that the bowel transit time was much faster in the natives with the high-fiber diet, and their stools were three times as large as stools of the English settlers. The faster transit time meant that the bowel toxins were not in contact with the bowel as long and were eliminated faster, as were cholesterol and fats. Dr. Burkitt believed that extensive use of low-fiber, refined foods in the United States and European countries was the basic cause of so much bowel-related disease in those cultures. He advocated using fewer refined foods and more fiber in the diet.

Today, the National Cancer Institute recommends that Americans eat at least 20 to 35 grams of fiber daily. Some foods have both soluble and insoluble fiber, such as oat bran, apples, citrus, and dried split peas. Cellulose fiber, as in wheat bran and oat bran, prevents constipation as it increases the bulk of the stool by holding water and by attaching itself to cholesterol, fats, sugars, and other nutrients. An analysis of ten clinical trials published in the *Journal of the American Medicial Association* showed that a daily intake of oat bran can lower cholesterol by 2 to 3 percent on the average. Breast cancer has also been reduced in those who have increased the fiber intake in their diet. Water-soluble fibers (pectins and gums) bind chemically to bile acids, which are breakdown products of cholesterol, and eliminate them. To compensate, the body makes more bile acids by withdrawing cholesterol from the bloodstream, resulting in lower blood levels of cholesterol. Both soluble and insoluble fiber bind glucose-containing carbohydrates and slow the entry of sugar into the bloodstream, which may bring at least some relief to diabetics.

Taking too much fiber can cause diarrhea, gas, and bloating. However, most Americans get only about 10 grams of fiber daily with their present diets, so there is little chance of excess. Good sources of insoluble fiber include whole grains, some breakfast cereals (read the food labels), whole grain breads, fruit, and vegetables. Two of my favorites are brown rice and oat bran muffins.

I also recommend powdered psyllium seeds plus husks, which can be purchased at most health food stores. People who take this add a level teaspoon of the psyllium to three cups of cold water in a quart jar, put on the lid, and shake it well for ten seconds. Then, they drink it down, stopping only to take short breaths, because the psyllium–water mixture begins to gel soon. Those who don't like the taste add a half cup of pineapple juice or some other fruit juice, then add the water. Follow the drinking of the psyllium–water combination with an equal amount of plain water and drink that, too.

Law No. 8: Do Not Overeat

The healthiest people I have met in my world travels were the same weight later in life as when they were in their twenties, and some of them were over 120 years of age! In the United States, one-third of all adults and 21 percent of all teenagers are over-weight, which leads to many health problems. The average person in our country picks up fifteen to twenty pounds from age twenty-five to fifty-five. When the body is overweight, the heart has to pump harder; the circulation is slower; pressure is placed on the hip joints, knees, and ankles; and often the colon will prolapse from the extra weight, which, in turn, presses on the pelvic organs. People have less energy when they are over-weight. Often, self-esteem is lowered. It is best to leave that extra food on the plate when you are full. Eating at home is prefer-able, since restaurants often add oils and fats to their entrees.

Overeating can cause many disturbances in the body. When the digestive tract is heavy and overburdened with foods (especially low-fiber foods), it becomes sluggish and transit time is slowed. This causes constipation and increases absorption of fats, cholesterol, and bowel toxins. When the colon becomes overloaded with waste materials it cannot pass, toxic chemicals from the bowel begin to seep through the bowel wall into the blood and lymph, and this puts a burden on the kidneys and the skin. People with skin conditions sometimes have toxic colons. (Acne, however, is not caused by a toxic colon.)

We have too many overweight people in our country. This can be caused by overeating as well as incorrect eating. In this country, 29 percent of the diet is made up of wheat, which builds fat. Rye builds muscle. When a person is nourished with the proper nutrients and is living a happy life, then he will not need to overeat. If a person is overweight and wants to diet, she should not reduce intake of essential foods. One helpful strat-egy is to go on a reduced sugar and starch food program. Sugar, and starches that convert easily to sugar, signal the body to store more fat. Only those who have willpower of steel can lose weight by eating less.

We should always choose good foods to eat. When visiting friends or traveling, plan in advance how you are going to eat to maintain your weight. It is also a good idea to fast one day a week. Food should never control us. We should eat only foods that will meet our need to have a chemically balanced body.

Some people have poor eating habits. They gorge themselves at times and starve themselves at other times. This upsets the body's metabolism. Some people do not get the nutrients they need during the meal so they binge on sugary snacks throughout the day. This can lead to serious health problems.

Weight reduction or weight control is very difficult without supervision. Some overweight people are finding it is very beneficial to follow a low-fat diet. If one consumes oils, they should come from whole grains and not be heated above 212 degrees Fahrenheit (the boiling temperature) in order to preserve any lecithin. A simple, sensible way of planned eating along with a challenging aerobic exercise program will bring most people's weight under control.

Law No. 9: Cook Without Water, High Heat, or Air Touching Hot Food

High heat, boiling in water, and exposure to air are the three greatest robbers of nutrients. Always cook at the lowest temperatures you can. It is impossible to get the best nutritional values from oils if they have been heated above 212 degrees Fahrenheit. Lecithin is destroyed in foods that are fried, cooked, or baked in ovens at a temperature higher than 212 degrees Fahrenheit. Boiling results in nearly a 50 percent loss of the nutritional value of potatoes, 40 percent of the value of cabbage, and 50 percent nutrient loss in apples.

Raw egg yolks are very high in lecithin, which keeps cholesterol in solution in the blood. Eggs may be boiled or poached to preserve lecithin, but frying destroys it.

Low-heat stainless steel pots with lids that form a water seal are the most effective means of cooking foods to preserve the greatest nutritional value. For oven cooking, glass casserole dishes with lids are fine. I approve of Crock-Pot cooking because it offers another low-heat, nutrient-saving means of food preparation.

Law No. 10: Bake, Broil, Roast, or Steam Meats

Poultry, fish, and red meat should be eaten sparingly—no more than three times a week. In my view, it is preferable to eat fish or chicken. If one eats red meat, it should be no more than once a week, and all the fat should be trimmed off. Never fry meats. The heat interface between the metal and the meat creates carcinogens. Baking, broiling, roasting, or steaming are more acceptable than frying because they preserve more nutritional values. Cook meat, poultry, and fish at lower heats for longer times to retain the most nutrients and flavor.

Avoid pork and fatty meats, and use only white fish with fins and scales. Salmon is permitted, even though it isn't a white-meat fish. Fatty meats lead to obesity and heart trouble. Beef is very stimulating to the heart, and I do not recommend using it. Eating meat more than three times a week can produce excess uric acid and other irritating by-products causing an unnecessary burden on the body. I believe that when we live a fast, hard lifestyle that includes having meat often, heart problems are likely to occur.

Law No. 11: Be Careful of Your Drinking Water

When we consider that every important function in the body requires water, we have to wonder why we don't conceive of water as more important than we do. All metabolic processes, respiration, digestion, assimilation, elimination, temperature regulation, circulation of the blood, the flow of lymph, and the intracellular environment require water. After each fetus develops in the water of its mother's womb for nine months or so, its soft, little body is 77 percent water. Water makes up 83 percent of our blood, 74 percent of our brain, and 22 percent of our bones. Perspiration is a natural cooling process that takes place when the body is overheated, in response to which two million sweat glands excrete moisture that is 99 percent water. We are cooled by evaporation. Water is essential to all of us, yet most of us don't drink enough. I believe most Americans are chronically dehydrated, some a little, some a lot.

The primary cause of constipation is dehydration—lack of sufficient water in the body. The majority of my patients over the sixty years of my active practice have been constipated, and I take this as evidence that most people don't consider water important enough to drink enough of it. You can tell if you are dehydrated by pinching the skin on the back of your hand; if the pinched skin stays up for a second or two (called "tenting"), you are dehydrated. Everyone needs to drink at least two quarts of water daily (more in hot weather or with heavy manual labor or sports like basketball) and needs to replace it. Eight 8-ounce glasses of water will do (two quarts); eight 12-ounce glasses of water are better (three quarts).

In his book *Your Body's Many Cries for Water* (Falls Church, Va.: Global Health Solution, 1998), Dr. F. Batmanghelidj writes, "If chronic dehydration is not recognized, and water intake isn't increased, risk of other diseases is greatly increased." I believe that. Fatigue is one of the symptoms of dehydration, and one can't help but wonder if dehydration plays some part in chronic fatigue syndrome (CFS), since Dr. Batmanghelidj considers it a contributing factor in other diseases. I believe doctors often overlook the importance of water intake.

Scientists say that only 10 percent of the fresh water in our country is fit to drink. When you consider that most countries don't even have that much good drinking water, you may begin to understand that water pollution at the global level is more than a minor problem. Most people could survive four to six weeks without food, but those same people would not last more than a week without water. Water is critically important for all forms of life, and pollution of good drinking water sources is a continuing danger—both globally and in our own country.

At home, I use reverse osmosis water, and when I go abroad I use bottled water or drink fruit or vegetable juices. I sometimes advise distilled water for my arthritis patients to help dissolve bone spurs. *Drink at least two quarts of good, uncontaminated water every day.* That amounts to eight 8-ounce glasses of water daily, not a difficult habit to get into. Most public water systems are highly chemicalized because groundwater sources are increasingly polluted. Juices and foods provide a significant amount of water but seldom enough. It is my opinion that high-quality drinking water, either bottled or reverse osmosis, is a must for good health. Dehydration leads to water imbalance in the body and constipation, processes that increase risk of several diseases. On hot days, drink more than two quarts of water.

LIVE ON THE SAFE SIDE OF MY FOOD LAWS

I worked out my food laws to make it easier for you to remember how to use food to stay healthy and avoid disease. Now that you know what to do, you are responsible for the nutritional basis of your health. Cut back on salt, and use natural herbs and spices to flavor your foods. A creative cook can make meals just as delicious within the boundaries of my eleven food laws as outside of them. If I had to add a twelfth law, it would be "Now enjoy yourself."

In changing over to a new way of eating, allow yourself a margin of grace. It isn't easy to change old habits or to give up foods that you now know are harmful to your health, but with patience and determination, you can do it. If you violate the food laws now and then, keep in mind the fact that it isn't what you do once in a while that affects your health, it's what you do most of the time. Just as one salad won't cure your arthritis, one chocolate bar won't send you to the hospital. Relax, but keep working on compliance. You'll enjoy yourself more as you come into harmony with nature and right living habits.

CHAPTER 2

HEALTH BUILDING BEGINS AT HOME

"Let your food be your medicine, and your medicine be your food" is a message carved in stone and left to us by Hippocrates (c. 460–370 B.C.), the ancient Greek healer credited with being the "father of modern medicine."

This ancient truth is as valid today as it was over two thousand years ago. Whole, pure, natural, fresh foods contain nutrients in such quantity and quality that they cannot be improved upon by processed or manufactured foods. The very essence of nature-cure healing is founded upon this truth. Nature inherently contains all the necessary preconditions for health and vitality when left undisturbed. It is the tampering of man that upsets this balance and throws him into states of disease.

Quality food is the first line of defense, the foundation upon which vibrant health and well-being are built. The literature supportive of this claim is abundant. In all cases, processing of any kind, especially the application of heat, destroys food values. There are very delicate essences present in fully ripened food grown on rich organic soil that can only be appreciated when eaten in the fresh, raw state.

DR. JENSEN'S HEALTH AND HARMONY FOOD REGIMEN

The best daily diet format, as described in Food Law No. 4 (see chapter 1), is two different fruits, at least four to six vegetables, one protein, and one starch, with fruit or vegetable juices between meals. Eat at least two garden salads a day. Sixty percent of the food you eat daily should be raw. I designed this Health and Harmony Food Regimen as a result of my work with thousands of people who came to my clinics, where I worked and taught classes on nutrition for over sixty years. I saw many people rebuild their health and regain their strength on this program. If you will make a habit of applying the following food regimen to your everyday living, you will be pleased at how much better you will begin to feel.

RULES OF EATING

- Do not fry foods or use heated oils in cooking.
- Do not eat until you have a keen desire for the plainest food.
- Do not eat beyond your needs.
- Be sure to thoroughly chew your food.
- Miss meals if in pain, emotionally upset, not hungry, chilled, overheated, or ill. (Sometimes the digestive system needs a rest more than the body needs food.)

RULES FOR GETTING WELL

- Learn to accept whatever decision is made.
- Let the other person make a mistake and learn.
- Learn to forgive and forget.
- Be thankful and bless people.
- Live in harmony—even if it is good for you.
- Do not talk about your sickness.
- Gossip will kill you. Don't let anyone gossip to you either.
- Be by yourself every day for ten minutes with the thought of how to make yourself a better person. Replace negative thoughts with uplifting, positive thoughts.
- Brush your skin daily (see page 110).
- Use a slant board daily (see page 106).
- Exercise daily. Keep your spine limber. Develop abdominal muscles.
- Walk in grass and sand for happy feet.
- Do not smoke or drink alcohol.

BEFORE BREAKFAST

Upon rising and half an hour before breakfast, take any natural, unsweetened fruit juice, such as grape, pineapple, prune, fig, apple, or black cherry. Or liquid chlorophyll can be used. Or use 1 teaspoon of vegetable broth powder and 1 tablespoon of lecithin granules and dissolve in a glass of warm water. Between your health drink and breakfast, do the following: skin brushing, exercise, walking, hiking, deep breathing, or playing. When showering, start with warm water and cool it down until your breath quickens. Never shower immediately upon rising.

BREAKFAST

Consume stewed fruit, one starch, and a health drink, or two fruits, one protein, and a health drink. (Starches and health drinks are listed with the lunch suggestions on page 30.) Soaked dried fruits, such as unsulfured apricots, prunes, and figs, or fruit of any kind, such as melon, grapes, peaches, pears, berries, or a baked apple, which may be sprinkled with some ground nuts or nut butter, are good choices. When possible, use fruit in season.

Supplements can be added to cereal or fruit, such as sunflower seed meal, rice polishings, wheat germ, or flaxseed oil (about a teaspoon of each). Even a little dulse may be sprinkled over cereal, together with chlorella powder or broth powder.

SUGGESTED BREAKFAST MENUS

Monday
Reconstituted dried apricots
Steel-cut oatmeal
Supplements
Oat straw tea
(Add eggs, if desired, or sliced peaches and raw cottage cheese)

Tuesday
Fresh figs
Cornmeal cereal
Supplements
Shave grass tea
(Add eggs or nut butter, if desired,
or raw applesauce and blackberries)

Wednesday

Reconstituted dried peaches

Millet cereal

Supplements

Alfa-mint tea

Add eggs, raw cheese or nut butter,

or sliced nectarines and apple and raw yogurt

Thursday

Prunes or any reconstituted dried fruit

Quinoa* cereal

Supplements

Oat straw tea

or grapefruit, kumquats, and poached egg

Friday

Slices of fresh pineapple with shredded coconut

Buckwheat cereal

Supplements

Dandelion coffee or herb tea

Saturday

Muesli with bananas and dates

Supplements

Goat's milk

Dandelion coffee or herb tea

Sunday

Cooked applesauce with raisins

Rye grits

Supplements

Shave grass tea

Cantaloupe and strawberries

Raw cottage cheese

---

*Note: Quinoa, a high-protein cereal grain dating back to the Incas, can be ordered through a health food store.

Preparation Tips

Reconstituted dried fruit. Cover with cold water, bring to a boil, remove from heat, and let stand overnight. Raisins may just have boiling water poured over them. This kills any insects and their eggs.

Whole grain cereal. To cook properly with as little heat as possible, use a double boiler or wide-mouth thermos to cook your cereal. Add cereal to boiling water in thermos, allowing enough room for cereal to expand. Add supplements as desired.

LUNCH

Consume raw salad or, as directed, one or two starches, and a health drink. The raw vegetable salad may consist of any combination of the following: tomatoes, lettuce (use green, leafy types such as romaine—no iceberg lettuce), celery, cucumber, bean sprouts, green peppers, avocado, parsley, watercress, endive, grated carrots, grated beets, onion, and cabbage (sulfur foods).

Starches

Choice of two: yellow cornmeal, baked potato, baked banana (or dead ripe), barley (a winter food), steamed brown rice or wild rice, millet (have as a cereal), banana squash, or Hubbard squash.

Drinks

Choice of one: vegetable broth, soup, coffee substitute, raw buttermilk, raw goat's milk, rice milk, soy milk, nut or seed milks, oat straw tea, alfalfa-mint tea, huckleberry tea, papaya tea, or any health drink.

SUGGESTED LUNCH MENUS

Monday
Vegetable salad with tahini dressing
Baby lima beans
Baked potato
Spearmint tea

Tuesday
Raw salad plate with hummus
Steamed asparagus
Steamed brown rice
Vegetable broth or herb tea

Wednesday
Raw salad plate with guacamole dressing
Cooked green beans
Cornbread or baked Hubbard squash
Sassafras tea

Thursday
Salad with raw blue cheese dressing
Baked zucchini and okra
Corn on the cob
Two Ry Krisp® crackers
Carrot juice

Friday
Green leafy salad with olive oil, herb, and lemon dressing
Baked green pepper stuffed with eggplant,
millet, herbs, and tomatoes
Split pea soup or fennel tea

Saturday

Vegetable salad with health mayonnaise dressing

Steamed turnips and turnip greens

Cornbread

Catnip tea

Sunday

Vegetable salad with lemon tahini dressing

Vegetable-barley soup

Steamed chard

Baked yams

Chamomile tea

3 P.M.

Have a health cocktail, raw vegetable juice, fruit juice, or fruit.

DINNER

Enjoy a raw salad, two cooked vegetables, one protein, and a broth or health drink, if desired.

Salad Vegetables

Use plenty of greens. Choose four or five items from the following: leaf lettuce, watercress, spinach, beet leaves, parsley, alfalfa sprouts, cabbage, young chard, herbs, cucumbers, bean sprouts, onions, green peppers, pimentos, carrots, turnips, zucchini, asparagus, celery, okra, radishes, tomatoes, garlic, chives, jicama, mushrooms, fennel, buckwheat sprouts, and sunflower seed sprouts.

Cooked Vegetables

Choose two: peas, artichokes, carrots, beets, turnips, string beans, Swiss chard, eggplant, zucchini, summer squash, broccoli, cauliflower, cabbage, sprouts, onion, or any vegetable other than potatoes.

Drinks

Herbal teas, vegetable broth, soup, or raw vegetable juices (carrot, celery, parsley, beet, fennel—any combination).

Proteins

Once a week: Red meat. Use only lean meat; never pork, fatty meat, or cured or smoked meats.

Twice a week: Raw cottage cheese or any cheese that breaks.

Three times a week: Poultry, fish, and lean red meat.

Vegetarians: Use soybeans, lima beans, pinto beans, and other beans; sunflower and other seeds; nut and seed butters; nut milk drinks; raw cheeses that break; eggs; and tofu. Vegetarians must be aware that being a vegetarian is more than just a diet of cutting out meat. I believe that being a vegetarian must include a way of thinking and a way of life. Vegetarians can choose from the vegetarian foods listed in this program.

Never eat protein and starches together. Note how they are separated in this program.

You may exchange your noon meal for the evening meal, but follow the same regimen. It takes exercise to handle raw food, and it is well to take a walk or a swim after the noon meal. That's why a raw salad is advised at noon. If sandwiches are served, always have vegetables at the same time. If you have a protein at dinner, a health dessert is allowed.

SUGGESTED DINNER MENUS

Monday
Salad
Diced celery and carrots
Steamed spinach
Puffy omelet

Tuesday
Salad
Cooked beet tops
Broiled steak or ground beef patties with tomato sauce
Cauliflower
Comfrey tea

Wednesday
Raw cottage cheese
Cheese sticks
Apples, peaches, grapes, and nuts
Apple concentrate cocktail

Thursday
Salad
Steamed chard
Baked eggplant
Grilled liver and onions
Persimmon whip (optional)

Friday

Salad

Raw yogurt and lemon dressing

Steamed mixed greens

Beets

Steamed fish with lemon slices

Leek soup

Lemongrass tea

Saturday

Salad

Cooked string beans

Baked summer squash

Carrot loaf

Lentil soup

Almond tea

Fresh peach gelatin with almond nut cream

Sunday

Salad

Diced steamed carrots and peas

Tomato aspic

Roast leg of lamb with mint sauce

Apple tea

CHAPTER 3

SPECIAL HEALTH-BUILDING FOODS

The human body is a complex structure of billions of specialized microparts and electrochemical processes, constantly moving, flowing, and changing in the state of dynamic equilibrium we call life. The average lifetime of a red blood cell is 120 days, and when it dies, it is replaced by a new one. As long as we provide the body with the biochemical nutrients it needs, the various organs and tissues can rejuvenate themselves indefinitely, provided we eat the foods that contain the vitamins and minerals we need.

If the body is not given the biochemical nutrients it needs, cells break down and die before their appointed time. If it is given substances it can't digest, use, or completely excrete, they remain in the body as toxic settlements in the tissue, reducing the ability of some organ or tissue structure to do its job. We must have the right foods to build and sustain wellness.

I have spent over sixty of my ninety-plus years watching out for the keys to good health and long life, traveling throughout the world and keeping my eyes open for vital health secrets. I have spent many years in live-in health spa work, observing firsthand what foods and therapies did for patients with various health problems.

In my work, I often found that my patients had deficiencies in important chemical elements, particularly sodium, calcium, silicon, and iodine. Each recipe given here was developed for the specific purpose of replacing certain nutrients that might be lacking in the body in order to assist the body in rebuilding and repairing weakened or damaged tissues. The following are special health-building recipes that I have used with great success throughout the years.

BROTHS

Potato Peeling Broth

Potato peeling broth is high in organic sodium and potassium, which assist in restoring calcium balance in the body. These foods are particularly useful in bringing calcium back into solution in cases of arthritis and in taking care of sodium deficiency in underactive digestive systems.

POTATO PEELING BROTH

2 cups potato peelings	*2 cups carrot tops*
2 cups celery tops	*1 medium onion*
1 tablespoon vegetable broth powder	*2 quarts water*

Finely chop all ingredients, add to water, bring slowly to a boil, and simmer for 20 minutes. Strain off broth and drink one or two cups a day. Do not store longer than two days. Vegetable broth powder can be purchased at your local health food store.

Variation: Peel 2 medium potatoes (¼-inch-thick) and simmer peelings only in a pint of water for 15 minutes. Strain and drink only the broth. This is a potent broth for assisting elimination.

Veal Joint Broth

Sodium, which occurs naturally in certain foods, is an element I have used most successfully in dealing with many people who were suffering from arthritis and general acidic conditions. Doctors "measure" a patient's age by the suppleness of the joints, and suppleness is attributable to sodium, the "youth element," which keeps us youthful, limber, and active. Sodium's importance is widespread in the body. It keeps calcium and magnesium in solution, helps keep the blood at the right pH, and is active in the lymph system.

Deficiency of organic sodium can result in stiffness, rheumatism, gout, and gallstones. Veal joint broth is rich in sodium and is an excellent support for the glands, stomach, ligaments, and digestive system, and helps to retain youth in the body.

VEAL JOINT BROTH

Fresh, uncut veal joint	½ cup parsley
1 small stalk of celery	2 cups half-inch-thick
1½ cups half-inch-thick	potato peelings
apple peelings	1 large parsnip
2 beets, grated	1 onion
½ cup fresh or frozen okra	
or 1 teaspoon powdered okra	

Wash a fresh, uncut veal joint and put into a large cooking pot. Cover half with water, and add vegetables, apples, and greens, cut finely. Simmer all ingredients 4 to 5 hours. Strain off liquid and discard solid ingredients. There should be about 1½ quarts of liquid. Drink hot or warm. Keep refrigerated. Use within two days.

Special Broth

This is a recipe I developed specifically for those suffering with arthritis or arteriosclerosis. Capra Mineral Whey is high in sodium, which helps to keep joints and arteries loose and limber. (Capra Mineral Whey can be purchased from Bernard Jensen International, 24360 Old Wagon Road, Escondido, CA 92027.) The vegetable broth powder helps this drink taste delicious because it is made of a variety of dried vegetables, such as celery, tomato, pimento, parsley, alfalfa, spinach, watercress, and carrots. All of these vegetables contain organic sodium as well. The third dry item in this recipe is lecithin, which is a dissolver. Lecithin helps to dissolve hardened deposits in the veins, arteries, and joints.

SPECIAL BROTH

1 teaspoon Capra Mineral Whey	*1 tablespoon lecithin granules*
1 cup hot water	*1 teaspoon vegetable broth powder*

Dissolve ingredients in a cup of hot water, stir thoroughly, and drink.

MILK SUBSTITUTE DRINKS (NON-CATARRH-FORMING)

What can we use in place of milk? Most Americans have taken an extreme quantity of milk and milk products into the body over the years, especially while they have been growing up and forming the different systems in the body. Milk and milk products amount to 25 percent of the average person's diet these days. It is necessary to realize that such a quantity of one single food in our diet will crowd out the other lovely foods we should be using. It is vitally important that we find a substitute for milk, and I have found several wonderful substitutes. Most of these can be found in health-oriented supermarkets or health food stores. You can make some of them yourself.

Many supermarkets carry commercial brands of soy milk, rice milk, goat's milk, almond milk, and other substitutes for cow's milk. If you can't find time to make seed or nut milk drinks, I encourage you to try these interesting new milk substitutes.

For all catarrhal troubles, I suggest that people eliminate wheat, milk, sugar, fats, and salt from their diets. These foods often produce extra mucus in the body, which can be the basis for colds, flu, bronchial trouble, allergies of all kinds, pneumonia, hay fever, sinus infections, and asthma. Children and adults with serious catarrhal problems do extremely well—a noticeable improvement in catarrhal conditions can be seen in a matter of weeks—by giving up wheat and milk and by using these alternative drinks made from seed butters, sesame seed butter especially, and almond nut butter. Sunflower seeds also make very good butters. These drinks cannot develop catarrh and, therefore, make wonderful milk substitutes. You do not have to worry about the balance of chemical elements. All the calcium and growth elements are there that are necessary for a child to build a good body.

Sesame Seed Milk

I believe that sesame seed milk is one of our best health drinks. It is a wonderful drink for gaining weight and for lubricating the intestinal tract. Its nutritional value is beyond compare, as it is high in protein and minerals. This is the seed used so much as a basic food in the Middle East.

SESAME SEED MILK

2 cups water   *¼ cup sesame seeds*
2 tablespoons soy milk powder

Blend all ingredients until smooth. Strain, if desired, to remove seed hulls (if hulls have not been removed).

Variation: Add 1 tablespoon carob powder and 6 to 8 dates. Blend for flavor and add nutritional value using any one of the following: Bananas, date powder, stewed raisins, or grape sugar. After any addition, always blend to mix. This drink can also be made from goat's milk, rice milk, or soy milk in place of the water.

Other Uses for Sesame Seed Milk

Add to fruits, after-school snacks, vegetable broths, and cereals; or mix with any nut butter. Take twice daily with bananas to gain weight. Add to whey drinks to adjust intestinal sluggishness and with supplements such as flaxseed or rice polishings.

Almond Nut Milk

Use blanched or unblanched almonds (or other nuts). Soak overnight in pineapple juice, apple juice, or honey water. Use in enough liquid to cover the nuts. This softens the nut meats. Blend nuts and water for two to three minutes. Flavor with honey or any kind of fruit, strawberry juice, carob flour, dates, or bananas. Any of the vegetable juices are also good added to nut milks. A good commercial brand of almond nut milk, produced by Pacific Foods of Oregon, Inc., is now available at health food stores and some supermarkets on the West Coast.

Nut milks can also be used with soups and vegetarian roasts as a flavoring or to pour over cereals. Almond milk is a very alkaline drink, high in protein, and easy to assimilate.

Soy Milk

Soy milk powder (and now soy milk) is available in almost every health food store. Add 2 to 4 tablespoons of soy milk powder to one pint of water. Sweeten with raw sugar, honey, or molasses and add a pinch of vegetable broth powder. For flavor, you can add any kind of fruit, carob powder, dates, and bananas.

Keep in refrigerator. Use this milk in any recipe as you would regular cow's milk. It closely resembles the taste and composition of cow's milk and will sour just as quickly, so it should not be made too far ahead of planned use.

Pumpkin, Sesame, or Sunflower Seed Milk

The same principle is used for making nut milks and seed milks. Soak overnight, liquefy, and add flavorings. Use in the diet the same as the almond nut milk. It is best to use whole seeds and blend them yourself. However, if you do not have a blender, seed meal can be used. Seeds and nuts can be ground in an electric coffee mill. Use any seeds and nuts except peanuts. For nut or seed salad dressings, use the same process, but add less water.

NUT AND SEED BUTTERS

The blender will chop nuts in three to five seconds; grind them to a powder in a little more time or reduce them to a butter. Quick switches to "on" and "off" at high speed and a rubber spatula to scrape off the sides accomplish this. The longer you blend, the finer the butter.

Sesame seed butter can be purchased in a health food store in a raw organic form. If you desire to make it, you can grind the seeds in a coffee mill until they are very fine and add a small amount of sesame oil. Dry, powdered herbs such as basil, dill, and thyme can be added for seasoning. Almond butter can be made in the same way by adding almond oil instead of sesame oil. If one has a juicer, directions are included for making nut butters. Many nut and seed butters are now available commercially.

SESAME SEED SALAD DRESSING

½ cup raw organic
  sesame seed butter

⅔ to 1 cup water

¼ teaspoon dill

½ teaspoon vegetable broth
  powder

¼ teaspoon basil

¼ teaspoon thyme

Blend all ingredients until smooth. Serve as a dip (with less water) or a dressing (more water). Lemon may be added to taste.

GELATIN

Gelatin is 85 percent protein with a trace of calcium and is mostly derived from the joint material of bones. In Europe, people often use bones with no meat on them as a base for soups. They cook them slowly so that some of the gelatin comes out into the soup, and then they remove the bones. Meats contain uric acid, but gelatin contains no uric acid. This is the reason I do not believe in using meat in soups. However, the gelatin from the bones is very high in organic sodium (which holds calcium in solution and helps prevent arthritis). I recommend the gelatin sold at health food stores.

We are as young as our joints. When the joints begin to get hard and stiff, they say you are getting old. Gelatin not only contains the sodium that holds calcium in solution and reduces stiffness, but it also contains one of the most easily absorbed forms of calcium one can put into the body. Calcium is called "the knitter" and helps to keep our bones and teeth strong.

GELATIN MOLD

1 teaspoon vegetable broth powder   *1 tablespoon gelatin*
1 tablespoon cold water   *2 cups tomato juice*

Dissolve the vegetable broth powder in 1 tablespoon cold water and gelatin. Bring the tomato juice to a boil and add gelatin mixture, stirring well to dissolve gelatin. Pour into cups and let stand in refrigerator until set. To lose weight, eat 1 cup of gelatin before each meal.

POWDERED SKIM MILK GELATIN MOLD

½ cup powdered skim milk   ½ cup cold water

1 tablespoon gelatin   1 cup boiling water

  or 1 tablespoon agar agar   1 teaspoon pure vanilla

Mix milk powder and gelatin or agar agar in ½ cup cold water
to a smooth paste. Gradually add boiling water to dissolve.
Flavor with vanilla. Pour into cups and let stand in refrigerator
until set.

APRICOT PIE

1 cup pulped fresh apricots   ⅓ cup lemon juice

  (or soaked dried)   1 cup cottage cheese

1 tablespoon gelatin   ½ cup raw sugar

3 eggs (separated)   9-inch baked pie shell

Mix apricots with gelatin in saucepan. Beat egg yolks and add
to apricot mixture. Heat to boiling over low heat. Cook 2
minutes, stirring occasionally. Cool to lukewarm. Add lemon
juice and cottage cheese. Chill until mixture begins to thicken.
Beat egg whites until stiff. Add sugar. Continue beating until
sugar dissolves. Fold into apricot mixture. Pour into shell. Chill
in the refrigerator until firm.

PUMPKIN PIE

1 tablespoon gelatin   1 teaspoon vegetable salt

1 cup cold water   ½ teaspoon ginger

1 cup boiling water   2 teaspoons cinnamon (scant)

2 cups pumpkin, stewed, sieved   Brown sugar to sweeten

Graham cracker pie shell

  (see following recipe)

Soften gelatin in cold water. Add boiling water and stir. Add remaining ingredients. Pour into graham cracker pie shell and chill in refrigerator.

GRAHAM CRACKER CRUST

⅓ cup butter

¼ cup brown sugar

1¼ cups crumbled graham crackers

Melt butter and stir in brown sugar. Add crushed graham crackers and mix thoroughly. Spread mixture evenly over a 9-inch pie container. Press to fit dish. Chill in refrigerator until firm or bake in 400 degree oven until outer rim of crust begins to brown. Let cool before adding pie filling.

SOY VANILLA ICE CREAM

1 cup soy milk

1¼ teaspoons gelatin

1 egg

⅓ cup honey

1 cup whipping cream

1½ teaspoons pure vanilla

Blend milk, gelatin, egg, and honey on high speed in blender until thoroughly mixed. Pour into saucepan and cook over boiling water until milk makes a white foam around edge of pan and gelatin dissolves. Cook 2 minutes longer. Return to blender and add whipping cream and vanilla. Mix on fast speed until blended. Freeze to a soft mush stage. Blend again until light and creamy. Refreeze until firm enough to serve.

PEACH CREAM

1 cup cold milk

½ cup health ice cream

¼ teaspoon cinnamon

1 cup sesame seed milk

1 cup sliced peaches

1 tablespoon gelatin

Blend ingredients in blender with a few pieces of crushed ice until smooth.

SARAH'S DELIGHT

1 tablespoon gelatin	*5 to 6 comfrey leaves*
1 tablespoon cold water	*1 cup unsweetened pineapple juice*

Soften gelatin in cold water. Melt over boiling water. Add remaining ingredients and liquefy until comfrey is very fine. Pour into mold. Set. Turn out onto bed of bronze lettuce. Ring around with shredded carrot. Garnish with a spoonful of cream dressing and half an olive.

CHEESECAKE

1 tablespoon gelatin	*1 lemon*
½ cup cold water	*Honey to sweeten*
1 cup boiling water	*1 pint cottage cheese*
	Graham cracker pie shell

Pour gelatin into cold water, add boiling water, and stir to dissolve. Add juice and zest of lemon, honey, and cottage cheese (sieve cottage cheese before adding), and mix well. Spoon mixture into graham cracker pie shell (see recipe on page 47) and refrigerate.

CORN ASPIC

1½ cups corn	*Dash of paprika*
2 cups milk	*1 tablespoon gelatin*
1 slice onion	*2 tablespoons cold water*
1 teaspoon vegetable broth powder	*¼ cup parsley*

Mix corn, milk, onion, vegetable broth powder, and dash of paprika in blender until very smooth. (Sieve to remove hulls, if desired.) Dissolve gelatin in cold water. Heat over boiling water to melt. Add to corn mixture and blend. Add parsley and blend until parsley is just chopped. Pour into mold and refrigerate. Serve on shredded lettuce with sliced tomato garnish.

BEET MOLD

½ cup raw sugar

¼ cup cider vinegar

1 teaspoon vegetable
broth powder

½ cup water

2 cups sliced raw beets

1 tablespoon gelatin

¼ cup lemon juice

Mix sugar, vinegar, vegetable broth powder, and water. Pour over sliced beets and steam until tender. Dissolve gelatin in lemon juice. Add hot juice from beets. Place beets in mold and pour juice over. When set, serve on endive and garnish with sliced avocado and hard-boiled eggs.

GOLDEN PINEAPPLE DESSERT

1 tablespoon gelatin

1 cup boiling water

½ cup raw sugar

1 can crushed unsweetened
pineapple

1 cup grated carrot

½ cup chopped cashews

½ lemon (juice only)

Melt gelatin in a little cold water, add boiling water to dissolve. Stir in sugar, add pineapple, grated carrot, chopped nuts, and lemon juice. Place in refrigerator to set. Serve with honey-whipped cream (1 cup whipping cream, 1 tablespoon honey, ½ teaspoon vanilla).

JUICES

Everyone should have some raw vegetable and fruit juice each day. Pomegranate juice is the greatest juice for cleansing the genitourinary tract. It can be very beneficial for bladder infections. There are many good juices, such as papaya juice, mango juice, and apple juice. Black cherry juice is very high in iron and one of the best juices for cleansing and nourishing the liver.

Beet juice is beneficial to the pancreas as well as the liver and gallbladder. Experiments made in Switzerland showed that beet juice could regress cancer in rats. Beet juice stimulates flow of bile from the liver and aids digestion.

Carrot juice is high in beta-carotene, which is particularly good for the eyes. It assists the body in building the melanin in the skin, which protects us from harmful ultraviolet rays. Parsley juice is high in chlorophyll, which cleanses and builds the blood. Celery juice is high in organic sodium, which helps keep calcium in solution. These last three juices can be drunk separately or mixed together. When we combine them, we receive more of a variety of vitamins and minerals.

Remember that a variety is recommended in all menus. Let us have a variety in the salad dressings, soups, juices, vegetables, and fruits that we have every day. Every fruit and vegetable has its own healing factors. They are grown in different soils, which contain different minerals. In getting a variety, we can be more assured of getting all the chemical elements the body needs.

HERBAL TEAS

All of the herbal teas are very helpful in a right-living regimen. Think of their value and try to relate to the particular problem you have. For instance, for weak kidneys, there is no reason why you should not use shave grass tea, parsley tea, or the kidney-bladder teas, such as KB-11. Following are just a few types of teas and their benefits.

Alfalfa–mint tea. This is a good tea that should be on everybody's shelf. Alfalfa is the highest-alkaline tea there is. Many people have overacid bodies, and this tea helps them to come into balance. The roots of alfalfa go as far as 25 feet into the ground, where they may pick up minerals and trace elements lacking in the topsoil. The mint helps dispel gas from the bowel and is an excellent digestive aid.

When I visited the Hunza Valley of Pakistan (known for the health and longevity of its people), the king invited me to his home and asked how he could get rid of his bowel troubles. I noticed that the king drank many cups of black tea daily with several teaspoons of sugar in each cup, which explained his bowel troubles. I went into the garden, where I found and picked fresh alfalfa and peppermint. I took this into the kitchen and made a lovely tea. I told the king to drink this in place of the black tea. He did and liked the new tea even better than the old one, and within one week, the king's bowel troubles improved greatly.

Asparagus tea. You can cook some fresh asparagus in water and take a half teacup of the water three times a day to help detoxify the kidneys.

Comfrey, mullein, echinacea, and fenugreek teas. If you have lung catarrh, these teas may be used two or three times daily.

Flaxseed tea. For eliminating toxic materials in the bowel, this is one of the great healing teas. It is useful for inflammation or irritations of the bowel, as well as for stomach ulcers. Flaxseed can be simmered in water for a few minutes and allowed to cool slightly before drinking. Flaxseed tea also makes an excellent soothing enema for an irritated bowel.

Hawthorn berry tea. This tea is high in the flavonoids and B vitamins. It is excellent for the circulation. It has often been used to restore the heart muscle wall as well as to lower cholesterol levels. It has been used successfully to treat heart disease, sore throat, and skin sores. It can be beneficial in relieving diarrhea and abdominal distention. Most people who are sick have poor circulation and fatigue. All sickness is a sign of stagnation in which the blood is not getting to all the organs and tissues as it should, and, therefore, not carrying the nutrients to the areas in the body where they need to go. Hawthorn berry tea is very beneficial to one who is ill because it supports the heart and improves the circulation so that the blood can carry oxygen (which gives energy) and other important chemical elements to all parts of the body.

Juniper berry tea. A good eliminating tea for kidney structure is made from juniper berries. Mash them, pour a cup of hot water over them, and let stand until the boiling water is just slightly warm. Drink this excellent tea for wonderful results. You may add a little honey, if you wish. Using this three times in twenty-four hours helps the kidneys to detoxify.

KB-11 tea (kidney/bladder). KB-11 is a tea made from eleven different herbs that are beneficial to the kidneys and bladder. These herbs help to strengthen and cleanse the kidneys and bladder as well as help them to release excess water. It is better to drink small amounts of this tea and not overdo it.

Oat straw tea. Oat straw tea is one of the best sources for silicon. In my clinical experience, I have found that oat straw tea helps to regenerate and strengthen the nervous system, rids the lungs of catarrh, and keeps the joints flexible. Its silicon content improves the hair, skin, and nails. It would be beneficial for a person with a weak constitution, who has weak tendons, muscles, and ligaments, to drink oat straw tea. Silicon has been called "the magnetic element" and is one of the great builders of the body. A spirited horse with a beautiful sheen to its coat has been fed a lot of silicon. Silicon helps us to feel energetic and alive. It helps our minds to work quickly.

Oat straw tea is one tea that must be boiled over a low heat for twenty minutes. It can even be used as a base for soups or cooked cereal grains. It is delicious and good for you.

Peppermint or chamomile tea. Both teas are good for stomach trouble.

FOOD AND SUPPLEMENT CONSIDERATIONS

- Reduce dairy product use. This includes milk, cheese, butter, and cream. Avoid using pasteurized dairy products. Use seed and nut milks and nut butters instead.
- Eliminate or reduce all *processed* sugar and other processed sweeteners such as corn syrup from your diet. Use substitute sweeteners *sparingly* such as whole raw honey, blackstrap molasses, maple syrup, and rice bran syrup.

- Increase the consumption of all vegetables and all fresh fruit.
- Eliminate all caffeine-containing foods or beverages such as coffee, sodas, black teas, chocolate, and so forth.
- Drink at least eight 8-ounce glasses of water each day in addition to or in place of juices, herb teas, and so forth.
- Eliminate refined table salt from your diet. Substitute sea salt, dulse, broth powder, vegetable seasonings, or herbs.
- Substitute brown rice, millet, rye, and yellow cornmeal for wheat. Cut down on starches and sugars.
- Use chlorella tablets or powder regularly to cleanse the body of heavy metals and environmental pollutants.

CHAPTER 4

WHOLE FOODS WITH SEEDS

his is probably one of the most important topics in food concepts. Nuts and seeds are the beginning of the next generation, and they are the foods of the future. Nature would not have the opportunity to carry on with a new generation without the procreative factors found in our mineral elements, enzymes, vitamins, and prostaglandins. Seeds carry the universal life force, and nature does a very good job of putting these things together for us.

We know that a seed contains the "embryo" of the plant within its protective coat and the stored food that nourishes the seedling as it develops into a new plant. Seeds take on everything possible from the mother plant. Very little air can penetrate the seed's protective coat. In fact, seeds buried in King Tut's tomb two thousand years ago were removed, planted, and grew into plants. Flower seeds two hundred years old were removed from the Spanish missions in Florida, planted, and beautiful flowers bloomed. Seeds are very important to us. When seeds from wheat and other grains are cooked in a microwave oven, they will not grow. The life force is destroyed forever.

Soil scientists have found that there are many minerals and trace elements in the ground, but they haven't gone so far as to find out everything they do in the plant. However, it is necessary to have a full array of the chemical elements needed for the seeds to grow into healthy, mature plants. All we need to do is give plants water, and the sunshine, air, and minerals all work together to grow them.

PROCREATION CENTER

There is a complex of biochemicals working together that makes seeds capable of developing the next generation. The seeds leave the mother plant and are ready to be planted themselves. They must have everything they need to begin the next generation. It is this procreative principle that is needed for the next generation's growth. Plants grow and develop a root structure, stems, and leaves. Limbs, stems, leaves, and fruit all carry a different type of chemical makeup.

Science is sometimes very crude in terms of its understanding of the finer forces in nature. Science hasn't done a particularly good job in finding out what nature really is and where the creative spark of life is that goes on to give the next generation its beginning and its reproductive ability. This procreative activity is also needed for reproduction of new cells when healing and reconstruction are taking place in tissue.

The root structure of each new plant is dependent upon the genetic inheritance from its parents. From that point, the new plant does the best it can from the nutrients available in the soil. They start building a seedling that grows into a tree with limbs, leaves, flowers, and nuts that man uses for food, for the building of his own glandular system, which will be used for developing his own next generation.

There's something we have to remember. Nature is very covetous in taking care of seeds. She put a protective coating on nuts and seeds that cannot easily be penetrated. Even with the strongest digestive system, the strongest hydrochloric acid content, we cannot break down the seed covering that nature puts on almonds, sesame seeds, and many other nuts and seeds. It is necessary to soak these nuts and seeds overnight to break down the coatings. That's why we liquefy them in a blender to make the nutrients more available for digestion.

It is important to prepare these foods properly in order to get their nutrients into the bloodstream to repair, rebuild, and renew the different cell structures in the body. It is not what we eat that counts, but what we assimilate into the bloodstream.

The whole seed is really where the "meat" of our life is contained. We must get to the heart of the seed, inside the hull, and it has to be crushed into such small particles that our digestive enzymes can break it down, change it, and get the micronutrients ready for the bloodstream to be delivered as food for the regeneration of cells. The body's cells must continually be regenerated. There's no part of our body that isn't visited by our blood, and our blood is only as good as the whole foods we eat. The whole seed is really where the beginning of life starts, where the new cell structure begins. This is the procreation center. Seeds are among the most important foods we can take into our body.

I believe the worst problem we have in this day is not properly educating people about cooking. Heat breaks up the molecular arrangement in a lot of our foods. We began cooking by boiling water, which was all man did early on, but now we fry foods with high heat. Food material is no longer "food" because of cooking. Cooking food with high heat, especially frying in fats and oils, causes more cholesterol problems than anything else I can mention. One of the greatest of all challenges today is to strive to overcome this particular sin of civilization.

Food value is destroyed with high heat. It destroys the natural enzymes people should have to promote digestion. The natural enzymes help other chemical elements put themselves in proper order, proper bonding, one element with the other, to engage the trace minerals in the body, and to give them the spark of life that allows a seed to grow. It's not just the mineral element factor. There is also a growth principle. Without enzymes, we will not have the new cell production we need.

Enzyme therapy may be the greatest breakthrough in our time. The way we cook our foods today, destroying enzymes and other nutrients, disturbs the molecular balance found in the natural, pure, whole, fresh foods we get from God's garden. This is one of the most important things I can tell you.

So many foods are being destroyed by preservatives, processing, frying, overcooking, canning in aluminum, and using the "five sins of civilization," which are wheat, milk, sugar, salt, and fat. By gaining the proper knowledge we need in food preparation, we can be healthier, happy people.

To have the finest family and the best of children, those who have the best start should think about this concept. If we are going to get away from rising doctor bills, we have to give our children the best health possible. It is from good seed that we raise good children.

All the organs, glands, systems, and tissues of the body are built from many nutrients. Among the most important are calcium, silicon, sodium, and iodine. Raw seeds, which new plants grow, tend to be relatively high in the first three minerals. Iodine is available in dulse, seaweed (the edible kinds), and in natural sea salt, as well as most seafood.

I was made aware of this while traveling through the Hunza Valley and staying with the king. There is a wonderful reflection from the mountains in the Hunza Valley. The mountainsides, in places, are green from oxidized copper. Copper is very important in building a good supply of red blood cells. We become anemic without sufficient copper in the blood (the recommended daily allowance [RDA] is 2 to 3 milligrams for adults). A significant amount of copper appears in Hunza-grown apricots. Hunza farmers were harvesting fruit and seeds from two-hundred-year-old orchards! Isn't this amazing?

When I visited the Hunza Valley in the 1950s, there were fifty thousand people in this valley with the most extraordinary health you can imagine. The apricot seeds were considered very important as a winter food in this valley, which was isolated from truck and auto access ten months of the year. The apricot seeds, to be edible, had to come from a good tree. They ate the inner seed of the apricot pit. These seeds were often sold or traded on the streets. It was a staple of the Hunza food supply, and these people were almost free of disease: no cancer, no heart disease, no hospitals, no doctors, no nurses—no drug stores. They had their health, in part, because of the apricot seeds. The only disease found there was goiter, due to iodine deficiency.

Most seeds and plants that have seeds are acceptable for consumption as food. Seeds contain lecithin, vitamin E, amino acids, minerals, and trace elements to support and maintain the nerves and central nervous system. Grape seed extract, for example, is a powerful antioxidant, perhaps fifty times more powerful than vitamin C. We must have the regeneration principles from these gland foods because the glands are very important in overall body functioning.

There are many seed-bearing plants we don't know much about yet. Leave them out of your food regimen. For instance, we don't know what would happen from eating avocado seeds or peach seeds; but we do know they would have effects. During World War I, peach pits were cracked and the inner seed was removed and used to filter out the gases intended to kill soldiers.

We should investigate seeds more deeply. We have mentioned only a partial list of the known edible seeds, but let me bring out one more point that is very, very important. Only a few decades ago, we couldn't even buy vitamin E. Where does vitamin E come from? It's not in the flesh of the fruit—it's in the seeds. High concentrations of vitamin E are found in wheat germ oil, safflower oil, and cottonseed oil. The germ is the procreative element that stimulates the seed to grow into the next generation. Without the germ, there could be no growth in seeds. And in the germ, along with the vitamin E, is lecithin, a phospholipid rich in choline that feeds the glandular system and the brain and nervous system. We cannot survive without the nutrients in seeds. We cannot live without vitamin E. We cannot survive without lecithin. And we can only get these nutrients from seeds.

The germ or life principle of seeds is missing, however, in hybrids. I'm sure you understand what hybrid means: "The offspring produced by crossing two individuals of unlike genetic constitution, such as different animals or different plants." I believe this is one of the reasons for all the reproductive problems in our civilization today. We cannot build a good regeneration system in ourselves on the foods most of us are eating without producing weak genes and inherent weaknesses. The orange had a hundred seeds in its original state. It was such a nuisance eating a fruit with so many seeds that the hybrid navel orange was developed. So the seeds were removed, and with that action, the hybrid fruit could not reproduce. Hybrid oranges with extra pulp and juice can be grown, but without the life principle that comes from the germ of seeds, we are not going to grow or have the best food possible. The glandular system of the human body will be lacking in essential supportive nutrients.

Some seeds contain the vegetable equivalents of natural estrogen and testosterone, the female and male hormones we humans need. Some seeds have more male hormone precursors and others have more female hormone precursors. Citrus seeds have both male and female precursors but are higher in the female, while date seeds have both but are very high in the male precursors. Thirty years ago, the Covalda Date Company started breaking down date pits and producing from its interior seeds a healthy powdered form that could be sprinkled on foods. This made possible plant-derived male hormone precursors in a form that could be used with meals.

How many people eat citrus seeds? I can tell you, almost no one. But, as previously mentioned, citrus seeds contain both male and female hormone precursors. Every person over forty should be using these. Men need a little of the female hormones also. They need to achieve hormonal balance by having both hormones in the proper proportions. These can be obtained from seeds, if we eat them. Mae West, one of my early patients, once said, "It's not the men in my life that counts, it's the life in my men!" This was said a little crudely, but she meant it. Mae West was very health minded. The strength in our generation as represented in our procreative ability is derived from nutrients like bee pollen, soy lecithin,

B-complex vitamins, and choline-rich foods. Zinc, vitamin A, pantothenic acid, vitamin E, cholesterol, folic acid, and the amino acid tyrosine are also needed to balance male and female sexual systems.

We are seeing many hybrid conditions in the human being today. We are bringing children into this world deprived of some or many of the important chemical elements. This would not be so if we spent more time understanding what proper nutritional support can do for us. For instance, with regard to some Down's syndrome children, the mother may not have had enough iodine to give the fetus. Calcium, iron, and folic acid are lacking in many mothers of children with birth defects. Caffeine, drugs, alcohol, and excessive fluoride intake are serious risk factors for birth defects. Many doctors recognize these dangers, but there is a lack of generalized agreement among health-care professionals concerning the need for advising women of childbearing age of such risks. As I have mentioned before, doctors are very busy people, and they are seldom taught enough about nutritional matters to have a good understanding of the risks and symptoms of excess or deficiency of the whole array of nutrients.

Our children being born these days may have unnoticed chemical shortages, which means there will be problems in their future. It is often difficult to identify deficiencies of certain trace minerals in the body. Unhealthy human beings are being born to parents with poor nutritional habits. Despite notices in restaurants and bars alerting pregnant women to the fact that alcoholic beverages may cause birth defects, our polls show that many pregnant women still drink alcohol and still smoke cigarettes. Malnutrition carries high-risk consequences that may lead to imbalanced antisocial behavior.

We are often not taught how to practice right-living habits in life. Unfortunately, those who try to bring right-living information to the public are often automatically opposed by a certain minority. When I lecture to my students, I sometimes ask if they feel they deserve the best, and they all raise their hands. But why don't we all take the best life has to offer? Shame on the doctors who haven't told their patients what's the very best for their good health. Health is not everything, but without it, everything else is nothing.

Following are lists of seed foods that build strong bodies. While we have given only a partial list here of the whole foods with seeds, it is far from complete, and there may be many more to come in the future.

WHOLE FOODS WITH SEEDS

Guava	Sesame seeds	Pomegranates
Pecans	Persimmons	Sunflower seeds
Almonds	Macadamias	Black walnuts
English walnuts	Pumpkin	Brazil nuts
Squash	Kiwifruit	Pine nuts
Watermelon	Hazelnuts	Cantaloupe
Hickory nuts	Muskmelon	Chia seeds
Honeydew	Coriander	Coconut
Loganberries	Flaxseeds	Raspberries
Dill seed	Blackberries	Cashews
Mulberries	Strawberries	Wild rice
Blueberries	Pistachio nuts	Papaya seeds
Celery seed	Quince	Figs
Okra	Beans	Prickly pears
Caraway	Cumin	Cucumbers
Kumquat	Anise	Soybeans
Mustard seed		

WHOLE FOODS

I want to remind you of my earlier definition of whole foods. Whole foods are foods to which nothing has been added and from which nothing has been removed. By implication, they should have been grown organically, in nutrient-rich soil, fertilized only with aged manure, compost, and other natural soil supplements. Whole foods, in some cases, may include foods like pineapple, coconut, carrots, avocados, and other foods that have some parts—seeds, hull, skin, husk, or greens—that are inedible. Milled grains, Rice Krispies, and potato chips are not whole foods. You can, however, cut up a potato, plant it, and the parts with "eyes" will grow.

Whole foods have the ability to reproduce their kind. Nature provides within whole foods all the nutrients to make a living plant grow and store carbohydrates. Seeds and nuts and foods like eggs and fish roe have all the right nutrients to build and support new life. This includes all the minerals, vitamins, enzymes, lecithin, nucleic acids, and natural oils it needs to make trunks or stalks, bark, limbs, leaves, stem, root or roots, fruit, and everything needed to make seeds to produce another plant of the same kind. The very nutrients contained in plants and seeds that give them their procreative ability are used in human nutrition to develop and sustain the sexual system and male and female reproductive processes. People need the nutrients in seeds, nuts, and whole cereal grains for healthy reproduction and healthy offspring.

Whole foods are complex in their natural structure, and it's very difficult for scientists to identify groups of nutrients with symbiotic relationships that should be eaten together. Food scientists have also tried to replicate chlorophyll, vitamins, and other nutrients in the laboratory, but they have only been partly successful. When laboratory-manufactured nutrients have been used on test animals and plants, there are often discernible differences in observed or analyzed effects as compared with natural nutrients.

I emphasize whole foods in my food regimen simply because they have the most nutrients in natural groupings that are most compatible with human needs. We cannot say of most manufactured foods that they will satisfy the nutritional needs of people as completely as their natural counterparts. We cannot say of hulled, milled, ground, and bleached cereal grains that their nutritional value even vaguely approaches the value of whole cereal grains. We cannot even say that preservatives added to an otherwise natural, whole food do not offer some risk to health—to some sensitive individuals or over an extended period of time.

Whole foods have been put together by nature in such a way that our highest technology is unable to identify, much less replicate, their capability of interacting with the human body to produce not just generic health and energy but that mysterious *elan vital* that gives life its touch of the miraculous.

Dr. William A. Albrecht at the University of Missouri demonstrated that food crops adapt, to a limited extent, to the kind of soil in which they are planted. Variations in weather can cause changes in plant development. Everyone knows that green plants don't grow at all in a dark room, no matter how rich the soil, and they don't grow well in dim light. They have to have full-spectrum light of a certain intensity. We've even made artificial light to imitate sunlight so that food crops can be grown indoors.

I knew Dr. John Ott, whose many significant discoveries about light and radiation are described in his book *Light and Health* (Old Greenwich, Conn.: Devin-Adair Publishers, 1973). In his distinguished career, he not only developed time-lapse photography but also pioneered studies of the effect of full-spectrum light on health. Dr. Ott invented artificial full-spectrum lights for homes and businesses, proven effective in preventing seasonal affective disorder (SAD). Tested in schools, this lighting has also helped students labeled as "hyperactive," who have attention deficit disorder (ADD). Currently, scientists following in the late Dr. Ott's footsteps are calling sunlight, or artificial full-spectrum light, an essential nutrient in human health.

It is wonderful to discover that the beautiful sunshine we take so much for granted is a vitally important part of our life. Fresh air, in much the same way, is also a pleasant and necessary part of our life. Photosynthesis, the basis of all plant life, requires sunshine, water, and carbon dioxide from the air to make carbohydrates, one of our basic food groups.

WHOLE FOODS

Tomatoes	Radishes	Celery
Broccoli	Peppers	Kumquat
Cauliflower	Lychee (litchi)	Loquat
Orange, seeds	Mango	Passion fruit
Peach	Pear	Banana
Plantain	Asparagus	Prune
Beets, greens	Alfalfa sprouts	Brussels sprouts
Cabbages	Carrots	Chard
Collards	Cucumber	Endive
Romaine	Leaf lettuce	Garlic
Green beans	Leeks	Onions
Kale	Chives	Mung sprouts
Lentil sprouts	Parsley	Mushrooms
Parsnips	Sweet potato	Soy sprouts
Rutabaga	Watercress	Turnips
Bamboo	Yams	Bok choy
Barley greens	Apricot, seeds	Whole grains
Cod roe	Eggs	Chinese peas
Plums	Figs	

CHAPTER 5

BRAIN AND NERVE FOODS

The brain, nervous system, and the glandular system are where the greatest catalytic and electrochemical activity takes place in the body. This is where enzymes are busy, speeding up and slowing down biochemical reactions, interacting with electromagnetic forces in the central nervous system (the brain) and the nerves throughout the body.

In my view, people *must* return to the natural foods, otherwise the spark of life that comes from the brain, nervous system, and the glandular system will gradually dim and go out. These systems are the ones from which the highest thought and creative achievement of humankind emerge. This is where our great classical music comes from; where the most wonderful poetry and drama are born, as well as the great works of art all over the world, which have awed men and women through centuries and many generations. This is where our senses and emotions interact. This is where we enjoy the scent of fine perfume. And these activities are all coming from the brain. Nerve signals from our sense organs terminate in the brain. There are integrative, evaluative, screening, and fine-tuning functions in the thalamus and hypothalamus. We "see" with the brain and the nervous system. We "feel" with our glandular system as well. The pheromones that exude from our skin influence subliminal reactions from those around us. Our conscious sensing of life, as it flows through us, is virtually a miracle.

The brain, nervous system, and glandular system require a certain nutritional input, and if we don't feed them properly, the functioning of both body and mind are impaired. Biochemicals, like lecithin and serotonin, are needed to form neurotransmitters that help control the passage of nerve impulses where one nerve joins another. Other biochemicals form neuroinhibitors. We find that two-thirds of our daily intake of blood sugar (glucose) is required to nourish the brain and nervous system. When there is inadequate blood sugar, we feel somewhat sleepy and tired, and we are slow in our thinking. Without sufficient glucose, brain and nerve cells die. Oxygen, equally important as glucose, must supply the needs of the brain's ten billion nerve cells, and this takes up at least 25 percent of the body's oxygen intake. We can understand why aerobic exercise is important, since it tones and exercises the lungs and brings in more oxygen than would be present for someone with a sedentary lifestyle. To supply this great need for oxygen, 20 percent of the blood supply is always in the brain, slowly flowing through the gray and white matter. The white matter of the brain is actually "insulation" for brain nerves, a sheath made of myelin, which is, in turn, made up mostly of cholesterol. The enzymes, which put the myelin sheath in position, must have copper, so copper is an essential brain element. Basically, the brain needs sugar, fats, lecithin, cholesterol, protein (in the form of specific amino acids), and oxygen. Since the brain is our "doorway" into what's out there in the world—it is the primary-care physician of the body and home of the soul and the spirit—it is wise to take the best possible care of it.

Vitamins and minerals needed for efficient brain functioning include the B-complex vitamins, folic acid, choline, inositol, and vitamins C, D, and E. The B vitamins work as coenzymes in hundreds of different tasks, including the metabolism of protein, the production of energy, and functioning of the nerves. Large doses of the B vitamins have relieved symptoms of senile dementia in patients in convalescent homes. Copper, folic acid, and inositol are all active in the care of the brain and nerves. Vitamin C works to protect iron, which brings oxygen to the brain via the blood, and copper, which works to maintain myelin sheaths. Vitamin D regulates cell functions, and vitamin E helps get oxygen to brain cells and protects memory. Indirectly, iodine affects the brain through its role in the thyroid gland, which regulates metabolism. Maybe that's why some people call seafood (high in iodine) brain food. Zinc is involved in over two hundred enzyme functions, including some involving brain activity. Chromium is believed to be needed by the brain, as is fluorine.

Most people don't have the slightest idea of how important it is to make sure that the brain, nerve, and glandular systems are fed and taken care of. (The same elements that feed the nerves also feed the glands.) The nerves and glands are extremely sensitive systems in our bodies. The hormones

secreted by the glands in microamounts are unbelievably powerful. The nerves and brain "steer the ship" and "plot the course."
All messages received by the body go to the brain, where they
are first screened for relevance, and then are passed along to the
appropriate response center. Motor nerves carry signals to the
body. Sensory nerves carry signals from the eyes, ears, nose,
tongue, and skin to the midbrain. Some ailments whose symptoms appear in the body have their source in the brain.
Epilepsy is a well-known example. Dyslexia is another.

At this time, it is impossible to tell how many of the so-
called symptoms of aging are due to poor nutrition, but I sus-
pect a great many of them are. I believe most older people are
more forgetful than when they were younger, and they forget
to follow a balanced food regimen. They might also be lacking
in funds to get healthy food. Generally, sick people are thirst-
ing for knowledge. They want to do the right things. My average patient wants to do the right things but doesn't know what
they are. Few people are able to live a healthy life on the
knowledge they have. Just a little study of healthy food habits
will help anyone find out how to live better with more available energy.

I believe there are very few people who know what it is to
really feel wonderful, to be well. The medical profession tells
us that four out of ten people who say they feel fine have a
chronic disease. I have never found a truly 100 percent "well"
person in my practice, which spans seventy years. The ultimate
is in reaching for that perfection. Without ideals or goals to
work toward, we can't improve our lives or our health. We can
be healthier as we go through life. It all depends on whether
we choose to live well. I say, "Go for it!"

FOOD FOR THE BRAIN, NERVE, AND GLANDULAR SYSTEMS

The following supplements, minerals, and foods in Table 5.1 are the most important to consider in healthy eating. They are a mixture of vegetarian and nonvegetarian foods.

Table 5.1. **Brain and Nerve Foods**

Gelatin	Sprouts	Caviar
Iodine*	Silicon*	Calcium*
Sodium*	Sulfur*	Phosphorus*
Lecithin*	Ginseng*	Ginkgo biloba
Chlorella****	Veal joint broth	Colostrum
Goat's milk	Goat cream**	Goat butter
Goat cheese**	Egg yolk**	Cod roe***
Turtle broth	Rice bran syrup	Vitamin B*
Clam broth***	Rice polishings*	Fish soup***
Germ of grains*	Cod liver oil***	DNA and RNA*
All seeds*	Nuts (hard-shell)*	Persimmons*
Shark fin soup***	Lady's slipper*	Avocado*
Seafood	Spirulina	

Dr. Jensen's *Forever Young* products:

    New Life Colostrum

    Your Youth

    Cleanse-It

    Di-Gest-It

    Maintain Wellness

* Foods for vegans.
** Foods for lacto-ovo vegetarians.
*** Foods for vegetarians who eat fish.
**** Chlorella (high in vegetarian B_{12})

CHAPTER 6

THE FOUR MISSING CHEMICAL ELEMENTS

There are four chemical elements I feel are missing in practically every patient who comes to me: calcium, sodium, iodine, and silicon. They are most prevalent in their expression and exhibition in the physical endeavors that people complain about. None of the chemical elements mentioned here is everything in itself. The body is a synthesis of eleven "macro" chemical elements and maybe as many as twenty "micro" trace elements. There's a lot of activity going on among these elements that we are prone to ignore in the flow of everyday life.

I studied the chemical elements with many teachers, but I was influenced most by my mentor, V. G. Rocine, a Norwegian homeopath. He taught me that the chemical elements have quite a story to tell. They are active in our lives—we live on them and depend on them. They belong to the dust of the earth; we take in that dust of the earth in the foods we eat. We're in a cycle, a temporary stage of having minerals entering and leaving our bodies. We have an ongoing exchange of the old for the new; as part of us dies daily, part of us returns to live daily.

New skin is made on the palms of the hands every twenty-four to forty-eight hours. We are being renewed all the time. What are we being renewed with? The answer is each of us is being renewed with the nutrients in the foods we have been eating in the last few days and with some nutrients from storage sites in the body. We determine what our bodies are being renewed with, for better or for worse—too often for worse.

CALCIUM

We need to target nutrients that our bodies need, not just foods we enjoy most. This cannot take place unless we know what chemical elements are needed, because each of the elements has a job to do. For instance, calcium is called "the knitter." It builds new bones and repairs broken bones; it "knits." There's three pounds of calcium in a healthy adult body, and we need 800 to 1,000 milligrams daily. If there is a shortage of calcium in the foods we use, the bones cannot knit. Calcium, when present in sufficient amounts, helps blood to clot, strengthens cell membranes, and serves as an electrolyte throughout the body. It works in nerve transmission. Calcium should always be taken with half as much magnesium. These two minerals are involved together in over three hundred enzyme reactions in the body. Calcium works with phosphorus, magnesium, and vitamins D and A to build bones (together with small amounts of other minerals like boron, fluoride, manganese, copper, and zinc). Osteoporosis can be slowly reversed at any age if calcium citrate is taken with small amounts of copper, manganese, and zinc. (Some forms of calcium, such as calcium carbonate, block the absorption of iron—calcium citrate doesn't.) Osteoporosis can be reversed faster in postmenopausal women if estrogen is taken, and even faster yet if regular exercise is included. Every patient I've taken care of has needed calcium. This is one of the most important elements in our bodies.

When a woman is pregnant, she needs more calcium. A new bony structure is being developed in the fetus in her womb, and it requires calcium. If there isn't enough of this element furnished from the mother's regular diet, then it will be taken from her bones. It will be taken from her joints, her teeth, and every large bone in her body. Back problems may begin to develop because of the lack of sufficient calcium. I have very seldom seen a woman who has delivered two or three children and has recuperated completely from the depletion of calcium. So it is well to know that calcium is probably our most important element. The best supplements are calcium citrate, calcium lactate, and calcium gluconate. If you are not using milk products, you may want to use supplements.

There are three other elements I feel are equally important: sodium, iodine, and silicon.

SODIUM

Sodium is the "youth element." Sodium keeps us young, active, limber, pliable, and able to jump for joy. We're not so settled that we can't move. Food-derived sodium keeps calcium in solution. When you go to the doctor and he says the joints are getting stiff because you're getting old, that's not entirely correct. Your joints are getting stiff because sodium is lacking in the joints. Many times people are told, "There's nothing you can do for this." All that most doctors offer are drugs to relieve your pain. When food sodium is lacking in the body, table salt and commercial acid neutralizers are not good substitutes. Food sodium can do a much better job. Sodium is stored mostly in the stomach wall, joints, and lymph, and these three areas cause the most trouble in older people. Sodium keeps calcium in solution, helps regulate blood pressure, takes part in nerve impulse transmission, and is used with the metabolism of carbohydrates and protein. We need 1.1 to 3.3 grams daily.

IODINE

Iodine is "the metabolizer." Every activity of every organ in the body is slowed down when the thyroid gland lacks sufficient iodine and becomes underactive (hypothyroidism). Many times, hypothyroidism is due to toxic materials. Even the bowel transit time is slowed because of the resulting reduction of metabolism. Every activity is quickened, on the other hand, when the thyroid is hyperactive (hyperthyroidism). In both cases, the thyroid gland needs more iodine because underactivity is caused by iodine deficiency and overactivity is consuming it. The thyroid needs adequate iodine, which is 150 micrograms each day.

Since every organ is affected by the lack of proper thyroid activity, we look to the thyroid as a very important organ in the body. Many of the patients I've seen had underactive body organs, and I tried to bring the activity to normal by treating the thyroid gland. Ninety percent of my patients, after the age of forty-five to fifty—both men and women—had hypothyroidism. This is why iodine is one of those chemical elements so necessary in getting a body well.

SILICON

Silicon is called "the magnetic element," maybe because of its use in computers. Silicon is the second most common element, next to oxygen, in the earth's crust. In the body, silicon is a bone builder, possibly with the function of attracting calcium, magnesium, and other bone-building elements to sites where bone is supposed to be enlarging or elongating. Rocine always taught that silicon was in the hair, nails, and skin, and that it coated the outside of nerve sheaths. Scientists are only just beginning to show an interest in silicon. At this time, it has yet to be proven essential in the human diet. I believe we need at least 200 milligrams daily.

I always liked the concept of silicon that Dr. Rocine applied to people. He always said, "Silicon people love to dance." Silicon is also found in the ligaments, teeth, lungs, trachea, aorta, and tendons. I personally believe that silicon is also necessary for messages to travel from the brain to different parts of the body.

In mentioning these four chemical elements, I'm not saying they are the most important, but the most often found to be deficient. If I can get calcium, sodium, iodine, and silicon back into the bodies of sick people, good changes will come about. This is how I use the chemical elements to get people well.

Many times people ask why I use and recommend some of the animal foods. First of all, I am a strong advocate of complete nutrition. I tried the vegetarian way, even tried to approach it all from a spiritual standpoint, but I found that in my work, I was so busy and exposed to stress that I needed more than vegetables. I could not find all the elements I needed in just the vegetables.

Every truly spiritual person knows that you can't have a healthy spirit in an unhealthy body. In order to keep this body right, the proper chemical support is needed, otherwise we have no temple in which to work. The spirit is an immortal thing. The mortal thing is the body. We have to take care of it through foods that contain the macro chemical elements and the micro trace elements.

We are an endangered species today because of the chemical shortages in people. Even the spiritual person is not living on the wisest side of life by having vegetables in their normal form and not having the live enzymes in their raw state. We're not getting all the trace minerals we need. I have to say, it is very important to have the chemical structure right, otherwise our body is not an adequate temple for the living God. It is not a godly temple with a godly spirit.

The foods listed on the next page are separated into the four chemical groups, and should be included in your daily diet regimen for your health. This list is not complete, but these are the *highest* foods in each group.

FOODS HIGHEST IN CALCIUM

Eggshell tea	Calf's foot jelly	Cottage cheese
Bone broth	Caraway	Kohlrabi
Raw cow milk	Lemons	Nettles
Cauliflower	Celery	Cabbage
Goat's milk	Lettuce	Sheep milk
Kale	Sea lettuce	Curly cabbage
Black radishes	Egg yolk	Florida oranges
Raw skim milk	Raw cheese	Fish with fins
	that breaks	and scales

FOODS HIGHEST IN ORGANIC SODIUM

Dried apples	Fresh apples	Unpolished rice
Roquefort cheese	Beaten egg white	Collard greens
Black radishes	Strawberries	Swiss cheese
Romaine lettuce	Raw buttermilk	Swiss chard
Celery	Cabbage	Rennin
Olives	Goat whey	Whole rice
Anchovies	Gizzards (poultry)	bran muffins

FOODS HIGHEST IN IODINE

Nova Scotia dulse	Kelp	Sea bass
Quail	Savoy lettuce	Sea lettuce
Silver salmon	Lettuce juice	Baked potato skin
Green turtle	Turtle broth	Raw oysters

FOODS HIGHEST IN SILICON

Asparagus	Raw rice bran	Barley
Celery	Whole rice flour	Cooked brown
Cucumbers	Oat straw tea	rice
Oatmeal muffins	Alfalfa broth	Dandelion
Wild rice	Wheat bran tea	Whole rice broth
Horseradish	White onions	Strawberries
Onions	Mustard greens	Marjoram
Wild strawberries	Rice bran muffins	Steel-cut oatmeal
Parsnips	Seafood	Bell peppers
Soybeans	Beets	Horsetail (herb)

CHAPTER 7

THE FOUR ELIMINATION CHANNELS AND THE LYMPH DRAINAGE SYSTEM

THE FOUR STAGES OF DISEASE

All diseases go through four stages: acute, subacute, chronic, and degenerative. A genetically weak area of the body is often the initial target. The acute stage is the active stage of disease, usually accompanied by catarrh, fever, coughing, inflammation, and soreness localized in the body. Catarrh may issue from any orifice in the body as demonstrated by a running nose, coughing and sneezing from the throat and mouth, tears from the eyes, catarrh from the ears, diarrhea from the anus, and vaginal discharge. In the acute stage, the body is actively trying to resolve the inflammation that marks the onset of disease, and all organs are hyperactive to support the elimination.

The subacute stage is more serious. If the body fails to throw off the disease in the acute, running stage, the inflammation sinks deeper into the specific tissues involved, reducing the metabolic rate and creating a localized underactive condition in the tissues.

The chronic stage finds the body in a lower condition yet. This is where flu, colds, and hay fever turn into asthma and occasional bouts of pneumonia. This is where joint aches and inflammation turn into chronic arthritis.

The final, or degenerative, stage is very nearly the point of no return. Asthma turns into emphysema. The joints swell and grow; in this stage of arthritis, calcium spurs appear on the vertebrae and in the joints. Lumps and tumors are found to be malignant.

Much of the poor health in adults can be traced back to childhood conditions. Many children's problems, such as colds, flu, earaches, mumps, measles, and tonsillitis, should have been taken care of by natural means to prevent catarrh from being driven back into the body. Cleanliness, correct foods, stimulating activities, and pleasant surroundings with plenty of love will keep most children well.

THE FOUR PRIMARY ELIMINATION CHANNELS

The four most important elimination channels of the body are the bowel, the kidneys, the lungs, and the skin. The lymph system works with these four systems by serving as a "garbage collector" to carry metabolic by-products and accumulated waste from tissues to the elimination organs. All these eliminative systems get rid of about four or five pounds of waste per day in the normal healthy adult. If any one of these channels becomes overloaded or clogged and slowed down, there will be extra pressure on the others and an accumulation of toxic material in the body tissues.

When the elimination channels have too much work to do, they become inefficient. Toxins, instead of being carried out of the body, are forced into the bloodstream where they are circulated to all tissues. The genetically weakest organs and tissues, which have the least resistance to deposition, become repositories for much of these circulating toxins. I call these genetically weak areas "inherent weaknesses."

The body is always generating waste material as a by-product of metabolic processes. Other waste is derived from food residues, which are of no use to the body, including pesticide residues, artificial colorings and preservatives, and residues of drugs. Significant levels of toxins also accumulate in the body tissues as a result of environmental pollution, not only from air, water, and chemicals, which are consumed or contacted directly, but also from pesticide sprays and industrial wastes, which get into the food chain from the air, water, and soil to the plants, fishes, and animals that end up on our dinner plate.

The buildup of toxins in the body tissues and in the bloodstream is the cause of lowered vitality and disease. Intestinal stasis (alimentary toxemia), in particular, is implicated in a wide range of conditions including fatigue, headache, asthma, hypertension, degenerative ocular changes, arthritis, degeneration of the muscles, liver, kidneys, and spleen, and many forms of cancer. As a result of over seventy years of work with patients at my health ranch, as well as extensive research, I have come to the conclusion that the four elimination channels are vital to everyone's health.

Following is an explanation of these important systems. It is important for each person to realize the necessity to clear the elimination channels, flush out the toxic settlements in the body, and supply the proper nutrients.

THE BOWEL

The bowel is the most important eliminative channel, consisting of 20 feet of small intestine and 6 feet of large intestine. In the great majority of people, I have found that the bowel is the most underactive organ in the body. The purpose of the small intestine, with its fingerlike villi, is the digestion, absorption, and assimilation of foods. The large intestine is divided into four sections: the ascending, transverse, descending, and sigmoid colon. It removes excess water and prepares to get rid of its load. Regular bowel activity promotes health. An underactive bowel increases the burden of toxicity on other elimination organs and introduces toxic material into the bloodstream and lymph, and this material then settles in the inherently weak organs and tissues of the body. Organs most affected by bowel underactivity are the lungs and bronchials, kidneys, skin, liver, and lymph system. These organs become overloaded with toxic settlements, and this leads to underactivity and mineral deficiency. The autonomic nerve system tends to become irritated and less efficient. It should be noted that a toxic bloodstream due to an underactive bowel affects *every* tissue in the body, but it affects genetically weak tissue the most. When the colon becomes toxic and underactive, many illnesses can develop. We need to take better care of the bowel.

Millions suffer from colon disorders. Studies show that over half a million people in the United States suffer from ulcerative colitis or Crohn's disease—inflammation of the colon marked by abdominal pain and diarrhea. IBS (irritable bowel syndrome) is commonplace. Colorectal cancer is a serious disease that occurs in the colon or rectum. Next to lung cancer, it is the leading cause of cancer-related deaths in America. One hundred thirty thousand new cases of colon cancer are reported each year, and as many as fifty-nine thousand prove to be fatal.

Developing positive attitudes, and managing our lifestyles so that we have rhythm, balance, and harmony with nature are very important for maintaining regular bowel movements. Eating meals without stress is most important. We should take time to eat our food peacefully without television news reports that might upset our digestion. Have pleasant conversations during mealtime or eat in silence. Eat early in the evening so that you don't go to bed on a full stomach. At night, the body needs to be resting, not digesting food.

Pay attention to when the bowel needs to move, and do not wait. Let the bowel empty entirely. When one ignores the needs of the bowel, interference with other body functions eventually develops. Ignoring the call of nature too often can cause a loss of sensitivity of nerve endings in the bowel, making one unaware of the time for elimination and ultimately leading to frequent constipation. Never force or strain yourself. This could bring about ruptures, hemorrhoids, or other rectal problems. (Hemorrhoids are varicose veins caused by too much forcing and straining at the stool.) Appendicitis can be another result of chronic constipation. The appendix is a small fingerlike projection that branches off the large intestine at the lower right-hand side of the abdomen. It is primarily lymphoid tissue, which provides a defense against local infection. People who become afflicted with appendicitis have often been constipated for years. When the colon becomes blocked and clogged in the area of the appendix with old waste material that has not been eliminated, the appendix can easily become infected.

So, the colon is the most important elimination channel for us to take care of. Many intestinal disturbances can be prevented. High-fiber diets can help a great deal. Raw or lightly steamed vegetables and fresh fruits provide good fiber. All foods that are yellow in color are natural laxatives, particularly good for the colon. (These foods are usually high in magnesium, which directly benefits the peristaltic action of the bowel.) Yellow squash, yellow cornmeal, peaches, and pears are wonderful foods for keeping the bowel well. Whole grains contain fiber, which absorbs water, swells up, and helps keep the colon clean.

I often recommend alfalfa tablets because they are high in chlorophyll and fiber to cleanse the colon, and acidophilus, which puts good bacteria back into the intestinal tract. Chlorella powder or tablets are excellent foods for nourishing the good bacteria and cleansing the colon. Research has shown that omega-3 fatty acids can be beneficial in relieving bowel inflammation. Fish of many kinds are rich sources of omega-3 fatty acids. Prunes and prune juice can also be helpful in maintaining regularity or relieving constipation. Cascara sagrada is a gentle, natural laxative if you must use one. Avoid regular use of commercial laxatives, however, which weaken the bowel musculature and create dependency.

Try to avoid coffee as much as possible and teas that contain caffeine. A good substitute in the morning is a cup of warm water or an herbal tea. There are many lovely, healthful teas to choose from.

Constipation can have many causes and can lead to many other ailments. Its most frequent cause is dehydration—failure to drink enough water. We all need to drink eight to twelve 8-ounce glasses of water each day. It takes time and determination to develop new eating and living habits, but for the sake of colon health, it is well worthwhile!

Specifics for Colon Health

Foods: Papaya, liquid chlorophyll, chlorella, prunes, figs, spinach, sun-dried olives, chard, celery, kale, beet greens, whey, shredded beet, watercress, yogurt, rice bran polishings, kefir, and psyllium husks.

Drinks: Parsley juice, papaya juice, chlorophyll, carrot juice, potato peeling broth, whey, prune juice, water with bentonite clay, and 2 to 3 quarts of plain water daily (juices and tea don't count).

Vitamins: A, B-complex, B_1, B_2, B_6, B_{12}, C, D, E, F, K, folic acid, inositol, niacin, and pantothenic acid.

Minerals: Magnesium, sodium, chlorine, potassium, iron, sulfur, copper, silicon, zinc, and iodine.

Herbs: Papaya, alfalfa, aloe vera, peppermint, slippery elm, cayenne, burdock, comfrey, ginger, fennel, anise, and cascara sagrada.

THE KIDNEYS

There are two kidneys and they lie in the abdomen, underneath the liver on the right and the spleen on the left. They are bean-shaped organs about the size of a fist, each about 4 to 5 inches long and about 6 ounces in weight. The arteries that supply the kidneys lead directly from the aorta, which is the main artery from the heart.

The kidneys filter the blood and excrete excess water and waste products in the form of urine. Each kidney contains seventy miles of filtering tubules called nephrons whose function is to conserve water, glucose, and essential chemical elements, and to eliminate acid by-products of protein metabolism and other wastes from the blood.

The kidneys filter two hundred quarts of blood in twenty-four hours and excrete two quarts of urine. They protect and conserve blood volume, electrolyte balance, and the acid–alkaline balance of the blood, and they influence blood pressure and the rate of red blood cell production in the bone marrow.

Kidney disease affects millions of Americans, and kidney underactivity is relatively common. Underactive kidneys affect the bowel, lungs, skin, lymph, heart, blood pressure, autonomic nerves, and many other organs and tissues by increasing the levels of harmful acids in the bloodstream and by altering electrolyte balance. The most dangerous waste products are generated by the breakdown of proteins.

An important function of the kidneys is to regulate electrolytes and blood. The kidneys control the body's acid–base balance. When blood and body fluids become too acid or too alkaline, the urine acidity is changed by the kidneys to restore balance.

The kidneys produce various hormones that regulate the production and release of red blood cells from the bone marrow. Vitamin D is converted into an active hormonal form by the kidneys. When the blood pressure falls, an enzyme called renin is released by the kidneys to constrict the small arteries and help increase blood pressure. The kidneys also secrete an adrenal hormone that acts on the tubules to promote reabsorption of sodium and the excretion of potassium.

The kidneys, like the bowel, are very important organs of elimination, with other vital functions as well. There are a wide range of kidney disorders that affect thousands of people each year. Hypertension can be both a cause and effect of kidney damage. Glomerulonephritis occurs when the filtering units of the kidneys become inflamed. Kidney stones are usually caused by excessive concentrations of various minerals such as calcium or uric acid. Infections can occur in the kidneys when there is an obstruction (such as a stone or tumor) to the flow of urine through the urinary tract, leading to stagnation.

Specifics for the Kidneys

Foods: Watermelon, watermelon seed milk, pomegranates, apples, asparagus, liquid chlorophyll, parsley and green leafy vegetables, and lecithin. Raw juices are also excellent.

Drinks: Celery juice, high in organic sodium, keeps calcium in solution and helps prevent kidney stones from forming. Pomegranate juice helps maintain the correct pH balance in the kidneys to assist the kidneys in fighting infection. Parsley, black currant, beet, asparagus, and grape juices (drunk separately) each help promote the healthy functioning of the kidneys. Goat whey is another drink that is excellent for the kidneys, as it is one of the highest sources of organic sodium. It is also a good source of chlorine and calcium.

Vitamins: A, B-complex, B_2, B_6, C, E, choline, folic acid, pantothenic acid, inositol, and riboflavin.

Minerals: Calcium, potassium, manganese, magnesium, silicon, iron, zinc, and chlorine.

Herbs: Juniper berries, uva ursi, parsley, goldenseal, slippery elm, dandelion, marshmallow, and ginger.

THE LUNGS AND BRONCHIALS

The third elimination channel I would like to review is the lungs. The lungs are cone-shaped organs that fill most of the chest cavity. They are made up of branches (bronchioles) and clusters of air sacs (alveoli). The lungs oxygenate the blood and eliminate carbon dioxide, a breakdown product of carbonic acid in the body. The lungs are also involved in regulating temperature, acid–alkaline balance, and lymph movement. Underactivity of the lungs and bronchioles affects the bowel, kidneys, skin, lymph, heart, autonomic nerves, and every other organ and tissue in the body by increasing the level of carbonic acid in the bloodstream, reducing oxygenation, and increasing catarrh levels and general acidity. Lung underactivity is often associated with allergies, asthma, lymph congestion, catarrhal problems, arthritis, fatigue, acidity throughout the body, and lower metabolism.

We must take care of these vital breathing organs of life! Pregnant women, especially, should take special care of their health and eat a good diet, rich with the nutrients needed by the unborn child to build healthy tissues, bones, and organs. Many problems can be prevented.

When the lungs are healthy, they eliminate as much as two pounds of waste materials every day in the form of vapor. When the lungs are weak and clogged with toxins, they are not able to eliminate properly. Living in an environment with a high level of cigarette smoke or other air pollution can cause lung disorders. Breathing asbestos fibers, silicon, coal dust, or radioactive dust can cause lung diseases that are often fatal.

Catarrh, often in the form of phlegm and mucus, is the universal symptom of imbalances in the body, indicating disease-producing processes at work. It is often the first symptom to appear (fatigue is also an early symptom) and is the body's normal response to an excess of acids and mucus being developed due to tissue inflammation. Catarrh can be caused by a deficiency of the biochemical elements in the body, an imbalance or excess of them, or a toxic irritant in the body. Catarrh is derived from the Greek words *cata* (down) and *rhein* (flow), meaning to flow down. As long as it is allowed to flow, we know the body's natural defense system is working properly. Its presence often signals the onset of a cold, flu, or other elimination process. Unfortunately, the most common response to it is to take a drug to stop it.

Catarrh can occur in any part of the body, and since the lungs are filled with small, porous, grapelike sacs called alveoli, they are good collecting places for mucus to build up. What causes catarrh in the lungs? There are many reasons. When a person has been a chronic smoker for many years, the lungs become coated with the noxious substances nicotine and tar. The lung tissue secretes catarrh as a protection from the irritants that are there. In a normal body, mucus is made by goblet cells in the mucous membrane linings. This mucus lubricates and protects the sensitive tissue lining these parts of the anatomy. If germ life, foreign matter, or toxic substances enter the body, they are entrapped in the sticky mucus, which is eventually excreted from the body as catarrh-flowing mucus.

Catarrh can also occur in people who have certain allergies or sensitivities to foods, such as wheat and dairy products. The gluten in wheat products can damage the wall of the small intestine in sensitive individuals or stimulate catarrh in those who are simply allergic to wheat. Lactose intolerance and allergic reactions to milk are different problems, but both are resolved by switching to milk substitutes like soy milk, nut and seed milks, rice milk, and others. Many processed, denatured junk foods cause catarrh as well. Continued use of tissue-irritating, catarrh-producing food products eventually interferes with the metabolism of inherently weak organs and results in the deposition of catarrh and vulnerability to disease in those organs.

If a child who has inherited weak lungs is raised on "pasty," catarrh-producing foods, perhaps in an environment of cigarette smoke, frequent colds often develop. If the colds are suppressed by well-meaning mothers who give the child medications, the sticky catarrhal material will be pushed back into the tissues of the lungs along with embedded germ life, foreign matter, and any toxic accumulations. This condition can develop into pneumonia or worse. With antibiotics administered, the child may appear to be free from symptoms, but in fact, the catarrh has been suppressed to a deeper level of tissue in the lungs.

Many times, children or adults who have suppressed symptoms of running noses and coughs and are symptom-free of these particular conditions will still feel fatigued in their daily lives. The body, in its effort to free itself from the overload of catarrh and toxic material in the lungs, will progress into pneumonia, bronchitis, asthma, and, finally, emphysema.

Most people fail to realize the price they pay for suppressing catarrh. A cough, for example, is a natural reflex action to rid the upper bronchial tubes and lungs of catarrh. From the advertisements of some cough medications, we find they work by suppressing the cough center in the medulla of the brain, which is a center directly related to the lungs. Other drugs act to dry up catarrh in the body, inviting the development of abnormal tissue pathology wherever the dried catarrh exists.

What are the alternative ways to remedy lung diseases? In my work, I do not deal with disease at all. I work with the whole body.

Elimination of Catarrh

When we know there are biochemical deficiencies in various organs, we can use diet and nutrition in our approach to eliminating catarrh. There are two basic steps in getting rid of catarrh, and they both work together. Cleansing the body through fasting, juices, and bowel management is half the solution. Correct nutrition is the other half. We purify the body as much as we can and we strengthen it as much as we can. This assumes that we are changing food patterns and other habits that may contribute to or aggravate the catarrhal problem, because our goal is to strengthen the body until it can eliminate toxic accumulations through the reversal process and the healing crisis.

Rearranging Process

Dr. Constantine Hering's law of cure states, "All cure starts from the head down, from the inside out, and in reverse order as symptoms have first appeared." Each time we have built the body up through right nutrition, exercise, positive thinking, and rest to the place where it reaches a certain level of strength, a healing crisis occurs in which suppressed symptoms of disease return and catarrh is liquefied and eliminated. Depending on how chronic or degenerative the disease has become, it may take several healing crises to eliminate the old catarrhal deposits.

I have never had a person under my care for a year or more who did not notice better health, fewer colds, and higher well-being. Any who have experienced catarrhal discharges from any part of their body noticed definite improvement. Properly selected foods and herbs make a decisive difference in ridding the body of catarrh.

For taking care of the lungs or any other part of the body, a person must first achieve a clean bowel. When the bowel is clean, the other organs then have a place to dump toxic wastes. A person with lung troubles should live in a place where there is clean air. They should omit dairy products, white flour, white sugar, salt, fried foods, processed foods, and alcohol from their diet. All or any of these can cause allergies, mucus, and catarrh, which the person with lung disorders must eliminate.

Specifics for the Lungs

Foods: Eat raw salads, green leafy vegetables, and fruit. These foods help to cleanse the catarrhal condition from the lungs. Replace all milk products with soy, nut, and seed milks. Rice milk is also excellent. Recipes for making these are given in this book. Consume grains that do not produce catarrh in the body. These are yellow cornmeal, rye, millet, quinoa, and brown rice. If one eats eggs, it is best to take the yolk raw, boiled, or poached so that the lecithin within it will not be destroyed, since lecithin is destroyed by cooking above 212 degrees Fahrenheit. If one eats meat, it should be organically grown and very lean. It should be baked or broiled and eaten no more than twice a week. The same holds true for fish and chicken.

Also beneficial to the lungs are garlic, onions, leeks, turnips, grapes, pineapple, and eucalyptus honey.

Drinks: Celery/papaya juice, carrot juice, watercress/apple juice with ¼ teaspoon cream of tartar, rose hips tea, goat's milk whey, and herbal teas, such as comfrey/fenugreek tea.

Vitamins: A, C, D, B-complex, B_1, B_2, B_6, B_{12}, E, F, inositol, choline, bioflavonoids, folic acid, niacin, pangamic acid, and pantothenic acid.

Herbs: Echinacea, goldenseal, mullein, cayenne, comfrey, colts-foot, garlic, thyme, elder flowers, peppermint, yarrow, lobelia, and marshmallow.

THE SKIN

The skin is the largest organ of the body, weighing 6 pounds in the average adult and covering an area of 2 square yards. Its function is to protect the body from the environment and to eliminate some of the same toxins expelled by the kidneys. Sometimes the skin is called the "third kidney." The elastic nature of the skin is perfectly designed to guard the sensitive underlying organs or tissues against chemical or physical damage. It also protects the body against excessive sunlight and the invasive efforts of harmful bacteria.

The skin is a sense organ and one of our major contacts with the outer world. It is a mirror of our general well-being. When the skin is underactive and not eliminating properly, uric acid builds up in the body.

The skin has often been neglected in remedial measures as an important channel of elimination. An example of the importance of the skin would be the way it works as an elimination channel for the lizard. The Gila monster eliminates entirely from the skin. Lizards live in sunny places in order to facilitate the sweating process. On a cloudy day, a lizard will have a very foul odor because the toxins are not being eliminated properly through the skin.

Likewise, it is vital for the skin of a human to eliminate toxic material each day. When the skin is not working properly, the pores can become clogged and may be dry and scaly, with boils, pimples, acne, psoriasis, and so forth. An underactive skin puts a greater load on other elimination organs. On the other hand, when the bowel, lungs, kidneys, lymph system, and digestive system are sluggish, many toxins must then be eliminated through the skin.

There are a variety of skin disorders, including acne, warts, psoriasis, eczema, and skin cancer. Localized rashes may appear on the skin from exposure to chemicals such as paint thinners or insecticides. A rash can also appear when the body is attempting to rid itself of poisons it has held in the tissues. It is important to keep these areas clean. Stay away from chemicals, and allow fresh air to get to the affected areas. Most of these conditions can be relieved through a diet that will assist the body in cleansing the tissues and replenishing the nutrients that are deficient.

Specifics for the Skin

Foods: A person should eat plenty of fresh fruits and vegetables and avoid greasy foods. Foods that have been found to be specifically beneficial to the skin are raw goat's milk, black bass, rye, avocados, sea vegetables, whey, apples, cucumbers, millet, rice polishings, rice bran, rice bran syrup, and sprouts.

Drinks: Raw juices good for the skin include a combination of carrot, celery, and lemon, and a combination of cucumber, endive, and pineapple.

Vitamins: Pantothenic acid, PABA, C, A, B-complex, B_1, B_2, B_6, B_{12}, E, F, K, biotin, choline, folic acid, niacin, and the bioflavonoids.

Minerals: Silicon, calcium, fluorine, iron, phosphorus, potassium, sodium, sulfur, iodine, copper, manganese, zinc, and magnesium.

Herbs: Oat straw, horsetail, shave grass, comfrey, aloe vera, and burdock.

The most important chemical elements for the skin are silicon and sodium. Silicon helps to keep the skin supple and elastic and sodium helps to keep it soft and free from psoriasis and other types of scaling and flaking. These two elements are included in the foods and herbs that were mentioned, with significant concentrations of silicon being found in raw goat's milk, black bass, oat straw tea, and horsetail tea. Sodium is abundant in raw goat's milk, whey, and celery juice.

Skin brushing with a long-handled, natural-bristle brush is an excellent way to clean healthy or unhealthy skin. Vigorously brushing the skin for five minutes daily helps to rid it of excess oils, dead skin cells, and toxic waste being expelled through the pores. (Avoid brushing the face or nipples.) Calendula ointment is made from the marigold plant and is helpful for all types of bacterial or fungal infections of the skin around the mouth or region of the anus and for itching rashes. Small cracks in the skin, such as splits, chapping, and fissures that may occur on the lips, in the corners of the eyelids, on the finger, or on nipples, will usually heal quickly when massaged with calendula cream.

THE LYMPHATIC DRAINAGE SYSTEM: THE CLEANSING RIVER OF LIFE

The lymphatic system is a network of vessels that drain lymph fluid and carry it centrally throughout the body until it eventually reenters the bloodstream. It is part of the immune system and plays a major role in the body's defenses against infection and cancer. The lymph fluid is a very clear, thin fluid, and its mineral salts are composed of about 80 percent sodium. There are 45 pints of lymph as compared to about 14 pints of blood in the body of the average adult. The lymph carries nutrients to the parts of the body where the blood cannot go and carries away waste, emptying it into the bloodstream.

The following analogy may help to explain the way the lymphatic system works. When we had our ranch, we had a drainage sewer system. If it ever got clogged and backed up, we found we had serious trouble in our cesspool. We also had a wonderful little stream going through the middle part of the ranch that not only carried off excess water but also circulated the water, keeping it clean. When it was running with clear, pure water, one could almost drink from it and depend on it being pure at any time. However, when it rained, some of the drainage from the dairy farm next door would enter our stream. Our beautiful, pure stream became dirty, discolored, and infested with waste material. In other words, our stream no longer had the purity it had in the beginning.

I compare our lymph stream to that stream of water running through our ranch because the lymph stream is supposed to be pure when it travels throughout the body to the various tissues, but it picks up impurities from the tissues that drain into it. Lymph system tissue and organs include the tonsils, appendix, spleen, breast tissue, and thymus. Lymph is very important because it even circulates in the narrow spaces of joints and the lens of the eye, tissues not penetrated by the blood. Lymph is moved through its vessels by muscle activity, exercise, and breathing. Lymph system underactivity most often affects the tonsils, appendix, breasts, joints, autonomic nerves, and the elimination organs.

A major factor contributing to lymph system overload is weakness in the elimination organs. Infections of the tonsils and appendix are common. Unlike the blood, which has the heart as its pump, the lymph must be moved by body movement, and Americans get far too little exercise. When the lymph stream is not pure, the impurities will finally get to the joints and various parts of the body in the form of uric acid and catarrh, which can cause rheumatic problems. Lymph can also pick up toxic waste from an underactive bowel and carry it to other tissues in the body, causing localized infections, aches, and pains.

If the proper chemical elements are not delivered to the tissues, problems can occur. For instance, calcium is held in solution by sodium, and when there is not enough sodium, the calcium will come out of solution. When this happens in the vertebrae and joints, knobs or spurs will develop. Without exercise, the lymph cannot efficiently carry nutrients to the areas where they need to go. Lymph nodes are located along the lymph vessel pathways in the joints, armpits, neck, groin, and spine, where they are protected by the strongest bony structure of the body. They are concentrated in these areas because the most movement takes place there. The nodes filter lymph fluid and remove dangerous impurities such as dead red blood cells, millions of debris-laden white blood cells, chemicals, dyes, and cellular debris.

The lymph nodes in the lungs of people who live in large, smog-laden cities are often completely black from the soot they breathe with the air. Sometimes the lymph nodes swell because of an overload of catarrh and bacteria and can be quite painful. People with inherently weak lymph systems have "swollen glands" quite often. These people hold water in their tissues more easily than others and will display a puffiness (edema) in their face, hands, and feet. They may gain weight from water retention and have difficulty losing it.

The lymph must be kept clean and free-flowing like the stream at my ranch. When it is not kept clean, wastes build up in the body and underactive tissues become deficient in necessary chemical elements. Many of us are exposed to chemicals in our water and air such as fluorine, cadmium, lead, mercury, pollutants from automobile exhausts, and sulfur dioxides. All this material can slowly become part of our lung structures, and it must be eliminated.

Boils and pimples may appear on the skin when the lymph is overloaded with toxins. The skin then becomes underactive. An excess amount of catarrh will begin to be discharged from the body. It flows through the nose, vaginal tract, ears, tonsils, and appendix. Women can develop lumps in their breasts when the lymph nodes become clogged in that area. The lymphatic system is our most important drainage system. Lymph drainage is probably the most neglected body function in the healing arts today.

In many cases, the catarrhal discharge is suppressed by drugs, and it backs up in the body. Never stop a catarrhal discharge.

There is much a person can do to prevent lymphatic congestion. When one walks, they should walk quickly, taking in deep breaths and swinging the arms to squeeze the lymph nodes. A mini-trampoline (also known as a rebounder) provides excellent exercise for the lymph system. Skin brushing is also an excellent way to move the lymph.

A person with a congested lymphatic system should eliminate all wheat and dairy products from their diet. These foods become quite pasty in the body and can easily clog the lymph vessels.

Specifics for the Lymphatic System

Foods: Eat green leafy vegetables, watercress, celery, okra, and apples. Chlorophyll is very cleansing for the lymphatic system. Both chlorella and spirulina are high in chlorophyll and can help detoxify tissues. Watercress acts as a natural diuretic and assists the lymph in getting rid of excess fluids.

Drinks: Potato peeling broth and raw celery juice are high in sodium, which is necessary for nourishing the lymph system. Also good are blue violet tea, parsley juice, carrot juice, and apple juice.

Vitamins: A, C, choline, B-complex, B_1, B_2, B_6, biotin, pantothenic acid, and folic acid.

Minerals: Sodium, potassium, and chlorine.

Herbs: Blue violet, chaparral, burdock, echinacea, goldenseal, cayenne, and mullein.

Exercises: The rebounder is excellent for moving the lymph. Walking, swimming, dancing, hiking, skin brushing, and the slant board are all excellent for the lymph movement. Active exercise squeezes the lymph nodes.

CHAPTER 8

PHYSICAL EXERCISE

Exercise of the human body is essential to maintain optimum health. Sedentary lifestyle results in the loss of muscle mass, tone, flexibility, strength, and vitality. In addition, there is a loss in similar qualities for tendons, ligaments, and bone. Other tissues tend to atrophy, which leads to physical degeneration.

All nutrients are assimilated better when we exercise regularly. Heat generated by physical exercise is a crucial regulator of many bodily functions. Some of these include the removal of gaseous waste as a result of cellular metabolism, enrichment of blood with vital oxygen, the improvement of nerve communication and function, the increase of the number and size of blood vessels, the improvement of blood circulation, and more.

If all other health-building practices are followed but exercise is neglected, you will not have the best of health. Physically active people are generally more alert, happy, cheerful, helpful, and vital.

Walking or swimming half an hour daily provides the best all-around exercise. The legs must be used because they are the pumps that drive the venous blood back to the heart.

PHYSICAL CONSIDERATIONS

- Slant board exercises daily to strengthen abdominal muscles and bowel tone.
- Rebounder (mini-trampoline) exercises fifteen minutes daily to music. Increase to thirty minutes over one month's time.
- Sunbaths to promote vitamin D production. Expose body to sun daily ten minutes per front and back (twenty minutes total). Best time is between 10 and 11 A.M.
- Exercise of some kind is essential for your well-being. Rebounder, running, walking, swimming, bicycling, tennis, hiking, and so forth, on a daily basis for a minimum of thirty minutes. Work up a sweat and breathe deeply.
- Periodic spinal adjustments for delivering ultimate nerve force to the body, such as chiropractic or osteopathic adjustments.

SLANT BOARD EXERCISES

The slant board is one of the finest and simplest pieces of exercise equipment for helping to deal with any physical problem caused or aggravated by gravity, pressure, or stress of daily life. Slant boards can be obtained from many stores where exercise or gym equipment is sold. Slant board exercises can help alleviate such symptoms as a dropped transverse colon, senility (by getting blood back to the brain), brain anemia, fatigue, varicose veins, hemorrhoids, and so on. The slant board helps compensate for the pull of gravity on the various organs of the body. It consists simply of a padded board with fold-out supports to raise one end 18 inches above floor level, with straps at the high end to hold the ankles.

In every fatigued and tired body, the transverse colon begins to drop. The transverse colon is the softest tissue in the body. It is tied up on the extreme right side and on the extreme left side to ligaments that go to the spine. Eight out of ten people who complain of back troubles have a prolapse that is basically the root of their troubles, causing a pulling on the lower part of the back. The slant board helps correct this by allowing the transverse colon to move back to its natural position.

Further, the slant board helps relieve the pressure caused by the upper abdominal organs that have dropped and rested on the lower abdominal organs, such as the prostate, uterus, rectum, and bladder. Prolapse problems in the abdomen also can contribute to hemorrhoids.

⌒⌒ Special Note for Slant Board Users

Certain individuals should not use the slant board. Anyone suffering from any degenerative disease with a tendency to bleed should avoid the slant board. Instances of internal bleeding, high blood pressure, extreme obesity, and easy fainting (when the head is below the rest of the body) are among those conditions contraindicating the use of the slant board. Pregnant women should avoid using the slant board. If you have any doubts or hesitations about using the slant board, check with your doctor.

Suggested Exercises on the Slant Board

Always wait two hours after eating before using the slant board. Follow instructions for the exercises below carefully. You can feel relaxed, refreshed, and invigorated quickly by stimulating circulation to all parts of the body. Do not try to do too much at first. Take on more exercises gradually. Do not attempt exercises that might aggravate a physical condition. (See "Special Note for Slant Board Users" on page 105.)

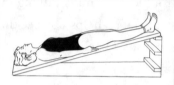

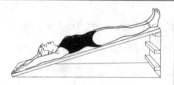

1. Lie flat on your back, allowing gravity to help shift abdominal organs into their proper positions and letting blood circulate to the head. Lie on board at least 10 minutes. This basic position should begin and end all series of exercises.

2. While lying on your back, stretch the abdomen by raising arms above head. Next, lower arms to sides. Raise and lower arms 10 to 15 times. This stretches the abdominal muscles and pulls the abdomen down toward the shoulders.

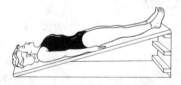

3. *If you are in great shape and under forty, you may be able to proceed safely with the following exercise. Otherwise, wait until you have exercised for at least two weeks, then proceed carefully, taking care to avoid excessive abdominal strain. Consult your doctor if you are uncertain.* Take a deep breath and hold it. Still holding your breath, alternately flex (contract) and relax abdominal muscles 5 times. You should feel your abdomen pressing upward toward your shoulders as you flex and feel it dropping down a little as you relax. Take a normal breath, then repeat the exercise 10 to 15 times, breathing normally between sets.

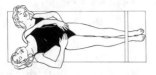

4. Pat abdomen vigorously with open hands. Lean to one side and then to the other, patting 10 to 15 times on each side. Reverse sides 3 or 4 times. Next, bring the body to a sitting position, using the abdominal muscles. Return to lying position.

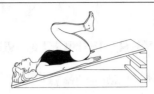

5. Holding onto the board, bring knees up toward chest. While in this position, (a) turn head from side to side 5 or 6 times, then (b) lift head slightly and rotate in circles 3 or 4 times. Reverse rotation. Repeat each set 2 or 3 times.

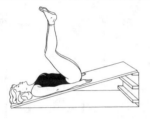

6. Holding onto the board, lift legs to a vertical position. Rotate legs outward in opposite circles 8 to 10 times. Change directions, rotating circles inward. Increase to 25 times after a week or two of exercising.

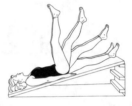

7. Raise legs to a vertical position. Keeping knees straight, slowly lower left leg to the board, then right leg. Raise each leg then lower each leg 15 to 25 times. Next, with legs in a vertical position, slowly lower both together to the board. Repeat 3 or 4 times.

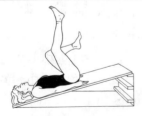

8. Raise legs to a vertical position. Bicycle legs in air 15 to 25 times. Do this at a slow pace at first, increasing speed gradually through the first week or two of regular exercise.

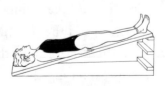

9. Lying flat on your back, relax completely, letting the blood circulate. Keep this position 5 to 15 minutes.

EXERCISING TO MUSIC

When doing any kind of exercises, one way to "lift the burden" is to have the kind of music you like playing, especially music with a good beat to exercise by. Different age groups will want to listen to their own kind of music. Lawrence Welk is one of the favorites for my generation. Rhythms such as heavy rock music seem to drain energy, but soft rock, some jazz, and other music with appropriate rhythms for exercise are acceptable.

REBOUNDER EXERCISES

Since aerobic exercises began growing in popularity a number of years ago, many exercise machines have become popular. Among these are indoor bouncing devices like small, short-legged trampolines that are easy on people with arthritis or overweight persons. Some are round, some are square, but all combine fun, convenience, and wonderful, vitality-building exercises. The great advantage of these bouncers over jogging or running machines is that they are springy and do not put such a jolt on the spine. Unlike outdoor exercises, they can be used rain or shine, and as often as you like during the day.

The legs are the pumps that drive the venous blood back to the heart, and the rebounder provides a wonderful way for working the legs to move the blood into all parts of the body, as well as exercising the heart and lungs. Air is drawn deeply into the lung structure, bringing a rich supply of oxygen to the blood cells, which are pumped throughout the circulatory system. This raises the vital energy at the cell level and rids the body of carbonic acid and carbon dioxide wastes. Using the rebounder is an excellent way to oxygenate the blood, improve circulation, exercise the heart and lungs, and get rid of metabolic wastes.

The lymph system, vital to health, is a network of vessels in the body very much like the blood circulatory system, except that it has no heart to act as a pump for it. Exercise is the only way we move lymph throughout the body since it is only through muscle contractions that the lymph is "squeezed" along through its vessels. The lymph is prevented from flowing backward by numerous one-way valves. To show the importance of lymph fluid, we have three times as much of it in our body as we do blood.

What does the lymph fluid do? It serves many functions, but its most important role may be as a key part of the body's natural immune system. Lymph nodes at the knees, groin, elbow, armpit, and under the jawbone make lymphocytes, which consume bacteria or foreign matter that gets past the neutrophils. Plasma proteins that form antibodies are also made in the lymph nodes. So, we see that one of the primary functions of the lymph system is to support the immune system, and we must keep it moving to get the job done. We must exercise to have a healthy lymph system, and we must have a healthy lymph system to have a healthy body. The lymph also functions to bring nutrients to the cells and to carry away metabolic wastes.

The spleen is the largest lymphatic organ in the body. Others are tonsils, adenoids, appendix, and breast tissue. The spleen acts as a garbage collector for worn-out red blood cells and other debris, while the tonsils sometimes pick up so much toxic material they become swollen and inflamed. If the lymph is not kept moving, toxic-laden areas can become sources of infection and inflammation.

The rebounder is one of the best ways to keep the lymph stream moving and avoid health problems.

The skin is sometimes called the "third kidney," due to its role in elimination, and when we exercise, the heat produced by the body increases the rate at which carbonic acid, waste salts, and water are eliminated through the skin and lungs. Using the rebounder is a convenient way to work up a light, healthy perspiration, getting rid of toxins and cleansing the skin pores.

Some have claimed the rebounder is a great help in losing weight, while others claim benefits to the eyes, particularly if certain eye exercises are followed while doing the body exercises.

So, considering all the advantages of the rebounder in terms of benefits to the lungs, heart, blood and lymph circulation, waste elimination, weight control, stress reduction, and possible improvement of vision, it is obvious that this marvelous miniature trampoline is one of the most versatile and health-enhancing pieces of exercise equipment we are likely to find.

OTHER BODY EXERCISES

There are other "exercises" that stimulate the body in different ways, and I consider these exercises extremely important for the health and well-being of everyone.

Skin Brushing for a Special Glow

The skin eliminates up to two pounds of toxic waste each day, depending on how much perspiration occurs. Uric acid crystals, catarrh, and various other acids are more easily eliminated when the top layer of dead skin is brushed away. Skin brushing helps get rid of uric acid to relieve the work of the kidneys, which normally get rid of two pounds of waste daily.

I believe that clothing made from synthetic fibers helps make us vulnerable to many diseases. It is important to realize we have to compensate for wearing clothing and for other unfavorable habits sanctioned by society. Clothes keep our skin from "breathing" properly. We do not allow our body to perspire in the fresh air often enough. We do not allow the sunlight to reach the body. To compensate for these shortcomings that cause skin—a major eliminative channel—to become inactive, I recommend skin brushing. Also, clothing is not, in itself, the only problem for the skin—it's the kind of clothing we wear. All synthetic fabrics, nylon clothing, panty hose, and so on, keep us from perspiring properly. Cotton and other natural fabrics absorb toxins and waste material from the skin. Synthetic materials block this elimination.

A *natural bristle* brush with a long handle should be used for skin brushing. *Never* use nylon, which will irritate the skin. Always brush dry skin, not wet, for two to three minutes each morning before a bath or shower or before dressing for the day. Rotate brush in all directions, avoiding the face. (A special soft brush may be obtained for the face.)

Kneipp Baths

The Kneipp bath, not including the herbal bath, is a wonderful water treatment for better circulation in the legs. It also relieves heart pressure. The bath consists of splashing through a 25- to 30-foot walk in cold water up to the knees, then a barefoot walk in grass or sand until you are dry. Do not wipe dry; if you do, you lose the value of the bath. The value is in stirring up your own circulation and in working to make sure the circulation takes care of the effects from the cold water. This exercise builds up the resistance in the body to take care of ordinary problems.

Another way of taking the Kneipp bath is with a common garden hose, without the sprinkler attachment. Run cold water, and starting at the farthest point from the heart—the right foot—move the water in a stream from the toes to the groin, then around and down the back of the leg to the ankle. Spray first the right leg front and back, two or three times; then do the left leg in the same manner. You should be able to count to six while running water up and down each leg.

This exercise is very good for circulation. Again, don't dry off. Run or walk until you are dry and warm. Do this exercise at least once a day.

CHAPTER 9

THE PREVALENCE OF MENTAL AND PHYSICAL CONDITIONS LEADING TO VARIOUS DYSFUNCTIONS IN THE BODY

We must always consider that diseases come slowly. We might develop a traumatic mental disturbance from years of worry or stress, and over time, this wears on the nervous system and produces nerve depletion. When we are constantly feeling rushed and have fear and worry in our daily routine, we disturb the adrenal glands. In the old days when people had tremendous fear of a wild animal, the adrenal glands pumped adrenaline to give the body energy for "fight or flight," and people used this adrenaline by either fighting or fleeing. The physical activity broke down the adrenaline to harmless chemicals that were easily eliminated. Now, when people are under tremendous mental stress, the body still produces adrenaline, but often their feelings are internalized. They neither fight nor flee from the situation. The adrenaline does not break down, and tissue damage results. In a business, people become stressed with work or their boss. In school, students become stressed by time limits and examinations. At home, spouses become stressed with each other or demanding routines with their children. Anger, stress, and fear are often held in for years. The adrenaline released repeatedly for years can cause serious internal damage. Whatever is not "expressed" becomes "depressed."

Many mental and physical health practitioners today are recognizing that mental and emotional conditions often have a direct effect on physical disorders. Research is showing that chemicals produced over years of time from unhappy emotional feelings can disrupt a body's physical balance and lead to disease. A stressed body, which does not get enough rest, will be much more susceptible to periodic colds and flu. Stress directly affects the immune system.

After years of sanitarium work with thousands of patients, I began to notice patterns in my patients who had emotional disturbances and how their ways of thinking and lifestyles had affected their health. I began to search for a better understanding of the links between emotional, mental, and physical health. Where should we start with all of these deficiencies that are developing in the body? How long is the period of time before mental disturbances begin to show physically? How should we look at them? How long does it take for water to drip onto a stone until it is worn away? It is hard to believe that it can take twenty years to start cancer in the body. How long does it take for emotional strain to break down a physical part of our body?

I have discovered that it's a matter of getting back to how we think and how we take care of our emotional feelings. We should ask ourselves, "Are we happy? Is our life flowing in rhythm, balance, and harmony? What can we do to create a healthy, happy life? Have we looked at the beauty of a flower lately? Have we been able to slow down properly? Have we been able to feel the warmth of the wind or a cold breeze that may cause a tingle in our toes? Are we aware that the mental and emotional life are probably the most important things to take care of?"

When we deal with the brain, we have to recognize that it is a physical organ. This physical organ depends on what thoughts and imaginations flow through it. We can have a godly attitude, a happy attitude, a deceitful attitude, or a fearful attitude, and these attitudes will have a direct effect on the type of chemicals the brain will produce and send to different parts of the body. You will feel this in your step and even in the marrow of your bones. It has been said so many times that God can only do *for* you what He can do *through* you. If you are blocked in your attitude with fears and doubts about life, then it is much more difficult to allow loving feelings to flow through. We can do much for our attitude by working with our internal thoughts and by rearranging our lifestyles.

My whole life has been based on finding a good healthy philosophy to live by. Without a good philosophy, a person cannot be well. There are two axioms I learned years ago that I am very much in agreement with. One is "We live on what we pour out." The other is "I don't feel sorry for the man who dies; I feel sorry for the man who does not live well." It isn't really how long we live, but how well we are while we are living! My mother used to say that you could lose all your money and you've lost a lot; if you lose your health, you've lost still more; but if you lose your peace of mind, you have lost everything!

In evaluating the many different people who have come to me, I consider the mental pressures they work under and evaluate them in the context of their attitudes and lifestyles. I find that many have developed nerve rings in their eyes and nerve depletion. They have broken down the good chemical nutrients in their bodies, namely lecithin, phosphorus, vitamin E, and vitamin B-complex. These mental and nerve nutrients are so necessary in our daily diets (or supplements) that we should all know how to keep from breaking down in our mental activities.

There are many symptoms, and all doctors know the importance of mind over matter. We control ourselves and organize our lives through the mind and the brain. More than $78 billion in prescriptions and over-the-counter drugs were produced last year in the United States. Most people use these medications properly, but a large percentage do not. In a recent year, the Substance Abuse and Mental Health Services Administration took a survey on drug abuse and found that over twenty-one million people over the age of twelve reported using one or more medical drugs (stimulants, sedatives, tranquilizers, and analgesics) for nonmedical purposes. These drugs are abused because they directly affect the brain and central nervous system. Many people make a living selling tranquilizers.

In Table 9.1 I have listed my personal estimations of prevalence of chronic dysfunctions, as I have found them, based on the patients I have worked with and observed. I didn't keep records of all these things, so my estimates are really "educated guesses."

Table 9.1. Prevalence of Chronic Physical Dysfunction Among Dr. Jensen's Patients

Eliminative Systems	Prevalence in Patients	Structural	Prevalence in Patients
Bowel	100%	Stress	65%
Skin	100%	Fatigue (tired tissues)	95%
Kidney	100%	Lower back	75%
Bronchi/lung	100%	Poor posture	40%
Hemorrhoids	100%	Hardened joints	50%
		Fingernail complaints	60%
		Rough skin/hair problems	75%
Circulatory System		**Toxemia**	
Circulatory impairment	80%	Drug settlements	100%
		Petrochemicals	50%
Anemia in extremities	80%		
		Nutritional	
Arcus senilis	80%	Low nutrient density	100%
Venous congestion	50%	Lack dietetic knowledge	100%
Poor oxygenation	50%		
Anemia	85%	Lack four most important elements: Ca, Si, I, Na	90%
Hardening of arteries	30%		
		Lack knowledge of risks of wheat, milk, sugar, fats, oils, and salt	85%
Glandular			
Low thyroid (over 45 yrs.)	80%		
Adrenal deficiency	75%	Dietary lack of proportion, variety, fiber, raw foods, combinations; overeating	85%

THE HOLISTIC APPROACH

We hear much about the holistic (or wholistic) healing arts these days, and this has come about as a reaction to doctors treating the symptoms only. No one ever has a disease of one organ while the rest of the body is healthy. When one part is affected, the whole body is affected. We have contributing factors, trigger symptoms, and reflex activities where the organ is poor, function is diminished, and the hormone or enzyme activity is depressed. Whenever this happens in any one organ, it affects every other organ. The basic concept of the holistic approach to treatment is that we are treating the whole person—mind, soul, and body.

Many times we do not treat the organ we should. The four elimination channels, I believe, produce many troubles with other organs, yet the elimination channels are seldom treated. If you look at the percentages of the prevalence of dysfunctions in the body that develop over a period of years to make a full-blown disease, we should start making changes early. We should start before deficiencies have developed in the various inherent weaknesses of the body. Start before clinical tests prove it to be serious. If we start early, before the ultimate breakdown, before one bad organ affects other organs, before we get into degenerative stages, then we can deal with the whole body and work with the holistic healing approach to set up a proper lifestyle to produce the highest well-being possible.

Some symptoms indicate that the body needs help, including sweating hands, gritting teeth, nose picking, bruising easily, dry skin, brittle nails, joint stiffness, bad breath, bowel bloating, constipation, dizziness, menstrual dysfunctions, and hundreds more. This means we have to take care of all organs and systems. This has to come from proper nutrition and supplying needed chemical elements. In your body's maintenance program, check which symptoms you may be experiencing from Table 9.2. There is a cause behind every one. Consult your doctor or nutritionist for the elimination of these symptoms. It's later than you think!

Table 9.2. **Prevalence of Emotional, Negative, and Harsh Mental Functions Found in Dr. Jensen's Patients**

Mental Condition	Prevalence in Patients	Mental Condition	Prevalence in Patients
Anxiety	50%	Lying	25%
Grief	20%	Greed	35%
Sadness	25%	Selfishness	35%
Disharmony	35%	Agony	40%
Impatience	40%	Misery	45%
Competitiveness	30%	Spite	20%
Envy	30%	Hate	30%
Cruelty	25%	Terror	35%
Brutality	25%	Mourning	20%
Stubbornness	25%	Sorrow	25%
Resistance	25%	Fear	35%
The executive's dilemma: serious, critical, analytical, exact	30%	Jealousy	25%
		Forgetfulness	25%
		People problems	50%

Note: These are faculties that people often think they need for success, but I have found they can break down the nervous system by 25 percent in the patients I have seen.

A HEALTHY MIND

I believe that it's impossible to be well without having a good philosophy. We have to know what it is to do the things we love to do, to eat nutritious foods, to get enough rest. We have to learn how to lay down problems. It's not the problems that cause us the trouble, it's how we look at them. We do not know how to go in the opposite direction when a serious negative thing comes into our lives. We hold onto it. We often hold grudges for weeks. We get involved in the past and carry it on into the future, spoiling every moment we go through.

In all my years of working with people, I have to tell you that you can't make it if you don't have enough love. Love is the key to life and happiness, but it must be a love that passes all understanding, a deep love beyond the physical realm. This love will carry you through and your five senses will be "fed" the proper nourishment through that love. It has a powerful effect on the physical body.

It's not just food that heals us, it's the mental and emotional aspects of our lives that make us who we are.

In order to heal yourself, you must become acquainted with Mother Earth, Brother Sun, Sister Moon, and our Father in heaven. We are a part of it all. Know who you are and learn where your place is. Be good to yourself. Let there be peace on Earth and let it begin with you.

These are the emotions that can get us into trouble:

Grief	Sadness	Disharmony	Impatience
Competitiveness	Envy	Cruelty	Brutality
Stubbornness	Resistance	Seriousness	Criticalness
Analyticalness	Exactness	Lying	Temper
Greed	Selfishness	Agony	Misery
Spite	Hate	Terror	Fear
Mourning	Sorrow		

Let's have a commencement exercise:

- Begin to begin . . . a new day
- Leave the past behind . . . where it belongs
- Out with the old . . . to make room for the new
- A new way . . . a better way

Let's begin with a new mental outlook, a new physical outlook, a new spiritual outlook. Begin each day with a whole, pure, fresh, and natural diet, outlook, and lifestyle. Take time each day to know what you like and what you don't like. Guide your life in the direction that's right for you. Be the captain of your ship.

Learn how healthy foods come from organic soil and grow from the ground up. Learn how to build a healthy mind and a healthy physical body. We are physical, chemical, electrical, emotional, mental, and spiritual human beings. We must work with the plant kingdom, the animal kingdom, the water kingdom, and all that dwells therein. We can develop our senses to a higher attunement to enjoy the sun, earth, air, colors, sights, and sounds. We can become responsible for our "ten acres," so to speak, on Earth and realize that we are in a new planetary millennium in which we must become conscious of living and working in harmony with nature.

LET'S STOP BREAKING DOWN

Nutrition, what we eat, is so important for nourishing the brain, nervous system, and the entire body. When our brain and nervous system are fed the foods they need, we can be stronger emotionally as well as physically. This is something to think about. The brain and nervous system are physical structures that have physical needs. When they are not receiving the proper nutrients, people become tired or depressed.

To heal ourselves emotionally, physically, and spiritually, we must change our attitudes to be more positive. There is such a thing as a healthy way of thinking, a healthy way of relating to people. At the same time, we should change our foods to those of the highest quality to feed our brain, nervous system, bones, muscles, skin, internal organs, and entire body.

Many people think they are eating nutritious foods, but often they are eating the same seven or eight foods every day. To get all the nutrients our bodies need, we have to have a variety. Very few people eat whole, nourishing foods with a nutritional food plan that will ensure variety in their daily diet. If we eat the same foods day after day, week after week, year after year, we are bound to have deficits of vitamins and minerals. Nutrient deficiency can make a person ill or chemically imbalanced.

It has been my experience, after seventy years of working in the health field, that when people get the proper nutrients from a variety of different whole organic foods, think happy thoughts, and live harmonious lives, their bodies will grow strong and healthy. Our bodies have a great capacity to heal themselves when given the environment and nutrients they need. It's also important to eat foods that are in season. Seasonal foods are much more nutritious for us than those that are grown by unnatural means when it is not the season for them. Our bodies are also more likely to create allergies when they are given the same foods over and over. Nature provides seasonal foods so we can vary what we eat. For example, tomatoes are in season and ready to eat in the summer, while pumpkins and many of the squashes are ripe in the fall. We should become aware of and cooperate with Mother Nature. She provides us with so many different nourishing fruits, vegetables, nuts, seeds, and grains. Winter is the time to eat foods that store well.

It has been my quest throughout all my travels around the world to endeavor to put together a food plan that would ensure a wide spectrum of foods that would supply the fiber, vitamins, minerals, enzymes, protein, carbohydrates, fats, and oils a person needs.

To review my recommendations in chapter 1, I recommend the following nutritional guide to be followed daily, unless you are on a tissue-cleansing program: six vegetables, two fruits, one starch, and one protein daily. Sixty percent of these foods should be eaten raw to ensure that we get enough fiber and living enzymes that are so valuable. Also, we should never cook with or consume heated oils. This changes the chemical matrix and causes them to be harmful to our bodies. Cold-pressed oils are better and should be used without heating, when desired in salad dressings. Cook in stainless-steel, low-heat cooking utensils. Never fry foods. Always use fresh, natural, pure, whole, organic foods.

I tell my patients and students there are five nutritional "sins" that cause problems if we eat a lot of them on a regular basis. These are wheat, milk, sugar, fat, and salt. When used in excess, these items can cause an overload to our systems and create catarrh, mucus, and even allergies. Of course, the more harmful things are caffeine, nicotine, alcohol, and other drugs. If you want to be healthy, these things must be omitted entirely.

It is important to realize that lowering our fat intake by 3 percent causes a 10 percent lowering of blood cholesterol. (When fatty foods in which cholesterol is initially balanced by lecithin are cooked at more than 212 degrees Fahrenheit, the lecithin is destroyed, leaving only the cholesterol. If the cholesterol had been balanced by lecithin, it would not be deposited on arterial walls.)

JACOB RINSE SUPPLEMENT

From near death due to cardiovascular disease, the chemist Jacob Rinse recovered his health enough to resume chopping wood and riding his bicycle ten minutes or so daily. He gave much credit to the following combination of nutrients, taken at the same time:

Lecithin	5 g
Vitamin C	500 mg
Sunflower seeds	12 g
Vitamin E	100 IU
Brewer's yeast	5 g
Vitamin B$_6$	40 mg
Calcium citrate	800 mg*
Magnesium	400 mg
Wheat germ	5 g
Zinc	10 mg

*Do not use bone meal or dolomite since the FDA has found lead and other toxic metals in them.

In 1998, over thirty-two million Americans were past sixty-five years of age. When the body's efficiency is diminished, as shown in Table 9.3, the processes that contribute to disease must be countered by a careful diet and supplement regimen, regular exercise, a healthful lifestyle, a cheerful disposition, and, if possible, tissue cleansing. To prevent disease and ailments, we must compensate as much as possible for metabolic slowdown associated with aging.

Be kind to yourself. Realize how important each and every human life is and that you are one of them. Recognize how the mind and body work together and how much more there is to each person than the physical alone. We are physical, mental, emotional, and spiritual beings. All parts of us need to be nourished—the physical brain with healthy foods; the emotional, mental brain with healthy thoughts. Organize your life in such a way that you can be happy and healthy.

If this seems overwhelming at first, begin with something small like using more whole, raw foods instead of denatured canned foods. Drink herbal teas or coffee substitutes instead of caffeinated beverages like coffee, tea, and colas. Caffeine is very damaging to the nerves, emotions, physical body, and brain. It can make you think you have lots of energy when your body could actually be exhausted and need rest.

Breathe more deeply, relax, find some time each day for yourself. When you are stressed, find out what the source is and try to work it through. Perhaps we don't have to "fight or

Age	Muscle Strength	Lung Capacity	Blood Cholesterol	Maximum Heart Rate	Kidney Function
25	100%	100%	198	100%	100%
45	90%	82%	221	94%	88%
65	75%	62%	224	87%	78%
85	55%	50%	206	81%	69%

Table 9.3. **Body Changes with Aging***

*Figures were taken from *Newsweek* magazine, March 5, 1990.

flee," but we just need to have a good talk with our spouse, friend, or boss. Perhaps we need to get a bicycle and ride it at the end of a hectic day at the office. Find what it is you need and do it! Realize that what you do today is paving the way for all of your tomorrows and, like a baby learning to walk, we must begin with a first step.

CHAPTER 10

THE REVERSAL PROCESS

When the health level improves as the result of changing to a right way of living, all tissues and organs cooperate in strengthening the weaker tissues in which suppressed materials have been stored. The stored toxic materials begin to be activated, moistened, and liquefied again, as if the body was being reversed to a previous condition of illness or disease. This is actually what happens in the reversal process. Just as we have unintentionally lived in such a way as to direct our body toward disease, we can now intentionally work our way back toward good health.

As we develop new tissue in place of the old, we gradually improve our health. When we reach a certain point in the reversal process, we become healthy enough and strong enough to trigger a healing crisis, which is nature's way of cleansing and restoring the body. I call this "replacement therapy"—new tissue in place of the old that is not satisfactory. When we reverse the process that brought on a disturbance or disease, we will eventually liquefy and eliminate the old toxic material and catarrh from the body, and the conditions that brought on the problem will be eliminated. *New tissue grows in place of the old.* This is true healing, and it is nature's way because tissue is restored with full recovery of function and activity.

HERING'S LAW AND THE REVERSAL PROCESS

Hering's law, which I mentioned in chapter 7, states that all cure comes from the head down, from within out, and in reverse order as symptoms first appeared. I use this homeopathic law as the basis for treating my patients.

This law means that as we follow the path of good health, every organ and tissue in the body begins to be strengthened and renewed. The stronger ones support the inherently weak tissues until a point is reached where the healing powers within the body suddenly begin to eliminate the stored-up catarrh, toxic material, old drug residues, and pollutants. This can be a little frightening because the healing crisis comes so abruptly and "acts like" a disease. But it is not; it is a cleansing process. Health is worked for; it is earned and it is learned!

THE HEALING CRISIS

When we begin to eliminate the old material, we have reached what is called a "healing crisis." This is the crowning reward of our efforts, a spontaneous and natural cleansing.

Unlike a "disease crisis," in which symptoms show that a toxic acid condition is developing in the body and the body is coping with the development of a disease, a healing crisis shows that old toxins are leaving, never to return if a person continues living right. Yet it resembles in every way a disease crisis, except that it lasts only a few days. The onset of the healing crisis marks the return of problems from the past.

Old Symptoms Return

There may be singly or in combination such discomforts as vomiting, diarrhea, fever, rash, skin eruptions, or discharges from any or all orifices of the body for about three days. Then it is gone, and the body is much cleaner. You will feel wonderful. This is nature's way of cleansing and healing.

During the healing crisis, you should rest as much as possible, taking only a little broth, vegetable juice, or chlorophyll and water now and then. This healing crisis comes when we have been following the right nutritional way and the new lifestyle path.

The main way to distinguish between a *disease crisis* and a *healing crisis* is that a healing crisis usually comes at a time when you have never felt better. One day you are walking on "cloud nine," and the next you are flat on your back, feeling miserable. This is usually a healing crisis.

This is an organized, proven system. It's no fly-by-night idea. This works, and everyone who follows this program will find out that it works. I have used it on thousands of patients, and those who have faithfully followed my directions have developed these healing crises. Patients have eliminated some of their oldest health problems, and many are now living in the best of health.

If the disease has gone too far and nature hasn't the ability to bring a return, then there is only one other way to turn, and that is conventional medicine—hospitals, drugs, surgery, and so on. What is essential to understand is that much can be done *before* we get to such an extreme stage.

IT TAKES ONE YEAR TO GET WELL

When a person is working to get well on a natural program, they should realize it will take approximately one year for the body to repair and regenerate. This is true healing and not just treating the symptoms.

In order to build a whole body, we need a variety of whole foods that are fresh, pure, and natural. In this way, we are assured a variety of nutrients that will nourish every cell in the body. Most illnesses are the result of a deficiency in one or more of the chemical elements.

At the end of a year of getting all the chemical elements necessary for health, a person will have a stronger reserve built up. A person should live through four seasons and build the body with the natural foods that are produced in each season. And just as we plant seeds in order for them to be harvested when they grow, we have to plant the seeds that are necessary to build good health in order to reap a harvest of wellness at the end of the "healing season."

CHAPTER 11

TODAY'S ENVIRONMENTAL PROBLEMS—WHY SUPPLEMENTS ARE NECESSARY

In today's world, there is air pollution, depleted soil, polluted waters, fruits and vegetables that have been sprayed with toxic pesticides, endangered species that are vital to our ecosystems, holes in our ozone layer, and genetically engineered foods. The amount of rich topsoil so necessary to provide the minerals needed to grow our plants and thus keep us healthy is eroding. Toxic waste dumps are accumulating around the planet, emitting noxious vapors that cause cancer and birth defects. Our immune systems are breaking down because we are eating mineral-depleted foods, breathing polluted air, and drinking water that has been treated with chlorine to kill the harmful bacteria. I must say, I don't believe for a minute that genetically engineered foods are okay to eat. They are *not* natural.

Are there any real and practical answers for humankind? What can be done to manage the rapidly deteriorating situation on our planet? What can one do to keep well while living in a polluted city? How does one cope?

For people who are obliged to live in large cities, there are powerful supplemental foods they can take to ensure that they get the nutritional chemical elements they need in order to stay well. Chlorella is one great example of these. Chlorella is an algae that is filled with all the vitamins and minerals needed for the health of human beings. It contains more chlorophyll than any other green plant, weight-for-weight. Chlorophyll plays a large role in keeping the blood clean. When the blood is not clean, then no part of the body can be truly healthy because the blood carries contamination to every cell. Research has shown many amazing benefits of chlorella.

At a conference on Bio-Regenerative Systems sponsored by NASA in the 1970s in Washington, D.C., Dr. Dale W. Jenkins of the Office of Space Science and Applications had this to say: "It has been amply demonstrated that chlorella can be used in a closed ecological system to maintain animals. The algae gas exchanger has the capability of efficiently supplying all required oxygen, rapidly and effectively removing all carbon dioxide, removing excess water vapor from the air, removing toxic odors from the air, utilizing waste water from washing, recycling water to provide clean water for drinking and washing, supplying food to animals to produce animal fat and protein." Because chlorella is so efficient at transforming sunlight into biological energy, chlorella could become a good fuel source in the future. Research has shown that chlorella is a good digestant for sewage, producing methane gas and fertilizer as by-products.

Chlorella, vitamin C, coenzyme-Q10 (CoQ10), alfalfa, carotene, and vitamin E are wonderful for getting rid of the dangerous free radicals that form in the body from pollution, radiation, toxic chemicals, and overexposure to the sun's rays or toxins in foods. Free radicals are electrically charged groups of atoms that can damage cellular DNA, accelerate aging, weaken the immune system, and invite infectious diseases. These supplemental foods have a chelating ability to bind with free radicals and escort them out of the body. They also nourish the body with important elements for the immune system.

Acidophilus is another wonderful supplemental food that is actually a friendly bacteria vital to our intestinal system. Acidophilus helps to protect against harmful bacteria in the colon.

Echinacea is an herb that helps to rid the body of catarrh and mucus that often collects in the lungs from breathing bad air. Vitamin B-complex nourishes the nervous system and helps one to handle the stress of the times. Calcium, magnesium, silicon, and phosphorus are minerals that are important to the health of the bones, teeth, skin, hair, and nervous system, and are also extremely important to the proper functioning of the immune system. People who live in cities should get a good water filter. They should buy organic foods, whenever possible, and eat foods that are pure, whole, fresh, and natural. As often as they can, they should go to the country for exercise and fresh air. They should take moments each day for contemplation and meditation to rest their nervous systems. Thus, there is much we can do to prevent disease, to keep our health, and to rebuild the health of planet Earth.

CHAPTER 12

CONCLUSION

I have spent a lot of time working in the drugless healing arts over the years, but I must say, there are no treatments that are worthwhile or complete without the use of nutrition. The role of the food shopper and cook is more important than doctors and surgeons in the building of health and in the prevention of disease. The cook can push loved ones into an early grave with a poor choice of foods. It is the responsibility of each cook to know all they can about nutrition, food chemistry, and food properties to keep the family well.

It is impossible to stay healthy on a wrong diet regimen. Almost all diseases are diet-related diseases. As long as we eat poorly, our doctors cannot cure us. If we eat right, we have little need for doctors. We have to learn how to heal ourselves. I have counseled patients, striving to guide and uplift them by building their health and teaching them that there is a right way and a wrong way to live.

In order to get well, we must exercise, and cleanse and purify our bodies. I have said many times, "You can't pour new wine into old bottles." In other words, we can't have new tissues until the toxic ones have been dealt with. It is important to exchange old habits for new and healthier ones. This is called replacement therapy. Replacement therapy can work in all phases of our lives. We can replace caffeinated teas with herbal teas, white flour with whole grain flour, sugar with honey, fried foods with baked foods, dour friends with happy ones, negative thoughts with positive thoughts, sedentary lives with exercise, toxic water with pure water, and polluted air with fresh air. Many people have lost all their reserves and are living in a deficit. When there are no more chemical elements to sustain the tissues, they become toxic and tired.

I have helped my patients by using a combination of proper nutrition, exercise, positive thinking exercises, water treatments, and other natural methods. This has been my method of treating my patients for many, many years, and it has proven to be very successful.

Despite the growing body of documented medical evidence that diet both causes and cures disease, nutritional awareness remains far from a twenty-first-century world ideal. Only about one-quarter of the 144 U.S. medical schools require instruction in nutrition. Even though half the medical schools offer it as an elective, only about 6 percent of students take one or more courses. By omitting the subject of nutrition, 25 percent of America's medical schools are not only perpetuating a nutritional "knowledge vacuum," they are sending out a negative message about the importance of nutrition in health as well. With our doctors ill-educated on nutrition, it's no wonder the public continues to lag in its own nutritional awareness.

The story of nutrition is not simply one of cure. It is also a story of life enrichment and well-being. Sadly, many people are living at only part of their full health potential, not really sick, but not truly well either. These people need to understand that the same foods that heal by rebuilding damaged tissue will enhance wellness by increasing the efficiency and energy level of underactive endocrine glands, and all other organs, glands, and tissues.

The basis for proper nutrition is found in the use of fresh, whole, pure, and natural foods. The number of calories in a meal means nothing unless they come from a proper balance of foods. If there is inadequate protein, the diet can cause you to become ill. If there is inadequate vitamin and mineral content, the same may happen. Even fats, in small quantities, are necessary for metabolism. Without the proper balance of a good variety of nutrient-rich foods on a continuing basis, good health cannot be achieved and maintained.

Wouldn't you like to wake up each morning feeling wonderful? Now you have the knowledge to make that a realistic option in your life.

INDEX